PEDIATRICS - LABORATORY AND CLINICAL RESEARCH

PEDIATRIC DIABETIC KETOACIDOSIS

RISK FACTORS AND PATHOPHYSIOLOGY, MANAGEMENT STRATEGIES AND OUTCOMES

PEDIATRICS - LABORATORY AND CLINICAL RESEARCH

Additional books in this series can be found on Nova's website
under the Series tab.

Additional e-books in this series can be found on Nova's website
under the e-book tab.

PEDIATRICS - LABORATORY AND CLINICAL RESEARCH

PEDIATRIC DIABETIC KETOACIDOSIS

RISK FACTORS AND PATHOPHYSIOLOGY, MANAGEMENT STRATEGIES AND OUTCOMES

STEPHEN C. DUCK
AND
JOSEPH R. HAGEMAN
EDITORS

New York

Library of Congress Cataloging-in-Publication Data

Library of Congress Control Number: 2015943272
ISBN: 978-1-63483-220-5

Published by Nova Science Publishers, Inc. † New York

CONTENTS

PREFACE

The future of persons with Type 1 Diabetes Mellitus is continuing to "look brighter" with the advent of biomedical technology. Nevertheless, the acute consequences of this disease remains a significant threat.

Diabetic ketoacidosis [DKA] remains the most serious challenge for primary care physicians and subspecialists caring for children and young persons with Diabetes Mellitus. Its prevention is possible only among those already diagnosed. Awareness of the etiology and clinical presenting signs among children of all ages is requisite for primary care and emergency department staff [Chapter 1]. While more likely to occur among those with Type 1 diabetes, a significant proportion of children with Type 2 diabetes are also at risk [Chapter 3].

Once diagnosed, the physician team must understand not only what biochemical imbalances must be corrected, but also what life-threatening complications must be avoided [Chapter 1]. The path through that "maze" is not yet fully interpreted; many choices remain as options, but each must be carefully evaluated.

Diagnosis among the very young is a challenge because of they lack self-awareness and clarity of signs and symptoms [Chapter 2]. Education of the primary care staff is critical and able to alter the incidence of DKA at the time of diagnosis.

Institutions that treat children and adolescents with DKA need an informed Emergency Department as well as Pediatric Intensive Care Facilities. Access to appropriate consultations, such as pediatric endocrinology, cardiology, neurology and neurosurgery are crucial.

The initiation of care is critical, and occurs invariably in the Emergency Department [Chapter 4]. Meticulous documentation of fluid composition and volume, insulin administration, vital signs and neurological state of well-being is essential. These will facilitate the transition to the appropriate in-patient service, whose task is to understand the biological impact of fluid rehydration and fluid flux, as well as hypocapnea, hyperglycemia and cranial perfusion [Chapter 5].

The current standards of care all but prevent most of the varied biochemical complications of "appropriate" care for persons with DKA. However, awareness of these possibilities is crucial [Chapter 6].

Yet, one complication remains unexplained and too often unpredicted, and it is devastating to the pediatric patient: cerebral edema. This complication, its prevention and treatment are discussed [Chapter 6].

Type 2 diabetes mellitus is continuing to increase in incidence and prevalence among all ages. Once thought to be "non-ketosis prone" diabetes, now persons undiagnosed or previously diagnosed do obtain DKA. They, however, have other unique medical requirements that must be applied to their treatment [Chapter 3].

Hyperglycemic hyperosmolar state is a complication no longer limited to adults with diabetes or children with Type 2 diabetes mellitus. While the incidence is fortunately lower than that of DKA, its outcome is potentially direr. Appreciation of the unique treatment requirements and guidelines are discussed [Chapter 7].

This monograph provides a comprehensive compendium to those caring for children of all ages with diabetic ketoacidosis, its related disorders and associated conditions.

In: Pediatric Diabetic Ketoacidosis ISBN: 978-1-63483-220-5
Editors: S. C. Duck and J. R. Hageman

Chapter 1

RISK FACTORS AND PATHOPHYSIOLOGY OF DIABETIC KETOACIDOSIS IN CHILDREN

Adebola Giwa*[*]*, MD, Payal Patel, MD, and Elizabeth Littlejohn, MD
University of Chicago Medical Center, Chicago, IL, US

ABSTRACT

Diabetes Mellitus (DM) is one of the most common childhood chronic diseases. The estimated annual worldwide incidence of approximately 65,000 children under 15 years of age is increasing at a rate of 3-5% per year [1]. DM is characterized primarily by destruction of insulin-producing pancreatic beta cells with resulting insulin deficiency or insulin resistance and a subsequent relative insulin deficiency correlating to type 1 or type 2, respectively.

A life-threatening complication of DM is diabetic ketoacidosis (DKA), which can be associated with polyuria, severe dehydration, electrolyte abnormalities, cerebral edema, and altered mental status. It is more prevalent in those with type 1 DM (29.4%) as compared to those with type 2 DM (9.7%) [2]. unfortunately, it is not an uncommon occurrence and overall, is the leading cause of morbidity and mortality in diabetic children [3]. Furthermore, DKA may be the initial presentation of type 1 DM. In these cases, the average frequency of diabetic children presenting with DKA is reported to be about 30% (15-67%) and is

[*] Correspondence to: Adebola.giwa@uchospitals.edu.

inversely correlated with the regional incidence of type 1 DM. This may vary based on age, family history, ethnicity, and geography. In those with known DM, the annual risk of DKA ranges from 1-10% [3, 4].

Due to the seriousness and increasing prevalence of DKA, it is important to understand the evolution of its development. Therefore, this chapter will address recent changes in risk factors and pathophysiology associated with the contemporary presentation of DKA.

Risk Factors

DKA as Initial Presentation

The primary risk factors that are associated with DKA differ in those presenting with DM for the first time, when compared to those with an established diagnosis. According to a large meta-analysis involving 46 cohort studies and more than 24,000 children in 31 countries, risk factors associated with DKA at diagnosis include: [1]

- Younger children, most noticeably younger than 2 years of age. A difference was still notable at 5 years but insignificant after 10 years of age. This is thought to be due to missed diagnosis given that with patients of this age group, physicians have a lower index of suspicion, the symptoms may be more subtle and difficult to distinguish from other more common illnesses, and there is a higher likelihood of quicker decompensation from the dehydration and acidosis [1].
- Delayed diagnosis due to diagnostic error during the initial visit with a physician and delayed treatment for more than 24 hours [1].
- Countries with low prevalence of type 1 DM due to an overall lower index of suspicion or decreased familiarity with the disease and its presentation [1, 2].
- Ethnic minority groups: the frequency of DKA in U.S. non-Hispanic white children was lower than Hispanics, Black/African-Americans, and Native Americans [1].
- History of recent febrile illness or infection, given that infections and other physical stressors activate a counter-regulatory response that contributes to increased insulin resistance and further metabolic decompensation [1].

- Lower family income: patients with a yearly family income below $50,000 were more likely to present with DKA than if greater than $100,000 [2].
- Lack of private insurance and no insurance: lack of adequate access to medical care and services can further delay diagnosis and treatment [1, 2].

Table 1. Risk factors associated with increased odds of presenting with DKA as initial presentation [1]

Risk factor	Odds ratio	95% Confidence Interval
< 2 yrs of age	3.41	2.54 – 4.59
< 5 yrs of age	1.59	1.38 – 1.84
Diagnostic error	3.35	2.35 – 4.79
Delayed Diagnosis	1.74	1.10 – 2.77
Lack of private health insurance	3.20	2.03 – 5.04
Preceding infection	3.14	0.94 – 10.47
No insurance vs Medicaid/public aid	2.84	1.16 – 6.93

DKA in Established Diabetics

The risk factors implicated in the frequency of DKA in known diabetics vary from those identified at initial presentation. These variables involve issues concerning appropriate management of diabetes, including both intrinsic and extrinsic factors, which could affect their homeostatic metabolic balance. According to a large cohort study of more than 1,200 children with known diabetes, some of these risk factors were found to include: [5]

- Increased age in girls: this could be attributed to body image issues since young adolescent diabetics often omit insulin injections to lose weight [5].
- Insulin pump therapy since failure leads to interruption of rapid/short-acting insulin in the setting of no long-acting insulin [4].
- Poorer glycemic control: those with a higher HbA1c or higher total daily dose of insulin [4, 5].

- Psychosocial issues including several psychiatric disorders, such as depression and eating disorders [4, 5].
- Lack of private insurance with subsequent limited access to medical services [5].

Table 2. Risk factors associated with increased risk of presenting with DKA in established diabetics [4, 5]

Risk Factor	Relative Risk	95% Confidence Interval
Higher HbA1c	1.68 per 1% increase	1.45 – 1.94
Higher reported insulin dose	1.40 per 0.2 U/kg/day	1.20 – 1.64
Underinsurance	2.18	1.65 – 2.95
Psychiatric disorders in males	1.59	0.96 – 2.65
Psychiatric disorders in females	3.22	2.25 – 4.61

PROTECTIVE FACTORS

Protective factors have also been identified with studies that have shown correlation with a decreased risk of presenting with DKA [1]. These include:

- Having a first degree relative with type 1 DM at time of diagnosis: this is likely due to a subsequent increased awareness of the presenting symptoms by experienced family members and a higher index of suspicion from medical providers given a positive family history [1].
- Higher parental education: with at least one parent having an academic degree (college diploma or higher) [1].
- Increased background incidence of type 1 DM: these areas are more likely to have providers with a higher index of suspicion; thus, they are able to diagnose and treat before symptoms evolve and develop too rapidly [1].

Table 3. Protective risk factors of presenting with DKA [1]

Risk Factor	Odds Ratio	95% Confidence Interval
1st degree relative with type 1 DM	0.33	0.08 – 1.26
Higher parental education	0.4	0.20 – 0.79
Higher background incidence of type 1 DM	0.715*	

* Correlation coefficient.

PATHOPHYSIOLOGY

Normal Response during Fed Fasting States

Metabolism is a multi-faceted process mediated by intricate processes involving various organs and biochemicals to ensure that the body's tissues have an adequate energy source to continue performing the processes of daily living. In order to do this, the body's energy, found in the form of glucose, lipids, and proteins, undergo a dynamic process of transitioning between utilization and storage dependent on the overall needs and resources available. Two key hormones involved in the process of maintaining euglycemia through a feedback system are insulin and glucagon, which are produced by pancreatic beta and alpha cells in the Islets of Langerhans, respectively.

During a meal (fed state), the body is in an anabolic state in which there is an adequate source of glucose for tissue utilization and an overall shift from producing glucose to storing it. During this state, glycolysis (the breaking down of glucose for ATP production) is actively occurring. In addition, glycogen (the body's main storage form of glucose) and lipogenesis are occurring at a brisk rate. Concurrently, since there is an adequate source of glucose, the processes involved in producing glucose including glycogenolysis, gluconeogenesis and fatty acid oxidation/ketogenesis are slowed or at a minimum [6]. At this time, insulin predominates and works to mediate both the movement and utilization of available glucose into the cells, subsequently lowering the serum glucose concentration.

After a meal (fasting state), the body is in a predominant state of catabolism in which relatively less glucose is available in the bloodstream and there is an overall shift into glucose production. During this state, glycolysis is blunted, and the storage processes of glycogen synthesis and lipogenesis stop.

Instead, the body must synthesize its energy source through gluconeogenesis and utilize its energy stores by glycogenolysis, lipolysis, and fatty acid oxidation/ketogenesis [6]. During this state, glucagon is relatively predominate and acts on the liver to activate the aforementioned processes of catabolism, thereby increasing the concentration of glucose in the blood.

Imbalance of Metabolic Homeostasis

Maintaining euglycemia, therefore, requires an elaborate feedback system involving insulin and counter-regulatory hormones such as glucagon, catecholamines, cortisol, and growth hormone. However, this balance is especially hard to maintain in diabetic patients who lack the intrinsic ability to make or respond to insulin (resistance). When diabetics have an imbalance in these regulatory hormones, with an inadequate circulating level of insulin associated with an increase in the counter-regulatory hormones or glucose, DKA may ensue.

In DKA, although there is an increase in the amount of glucose available, there is an inability for it to be taken up and utilized at a cellular level, leading to hyperglycemia and subsequent hyperosmolality. Without the appropriate amount of insulin, the body is unable to utilize the peripheral glucose giving the erroneous impression that there is a deficit. The body responds by shifting into a fasting state in a misguided attempt to produce more glucose. Subsequently, processes such as lipolysis increase, leading to ketone body (B-hydroxybutyrate and acetoacetate) production and eventually causes ketonemia, ketonuria, and metabolic acidosis. In addition, hyperglycemia and acidosis lead to osmotic diuresis, dehydration, and obligate loss of electrolytes with the resultant complication of this metabolic imbalance, or DKA [3, 7].

According to the 2014 International Society for Pediatric and Adolescent Diabetes (ISPAD) Clinical Practice Consensus Guideline Compendium, the biochemical criteria for DKA include [4]:

- Hyperglycemia (blood glucose > 11mmol/L; ~ 200mg/dL)
- Venous pH < 7.3 and/or bicarbonate < 15 mmol/L
- Ketonemia (beta hydroxybutyrate concentration > 3mmol/L)
- Ketonuria (>/= 2+; moderate/large)

Lack of Insulin

Between meals, the concentration of glucagon must be relatively higher than insulin to maintain the hepatic fuel production necessary to meet the body's energy needs. In DM, either the lack of insulin normally supplied by beta cells or increased insulin resistance, prevents the necessary influx of glucose into the cells, thereby preventing the body from achieving its fuel needs. In both cases, hyperglycemia develops due to the inability of intravascular glucose to enter the cells. In addition, the deficit "tricks" the body into believing that there is no insulin because there is no uptake of glucose. The body then, in turn, upregulates the production of glucagon as a counter-regulatory mechanism in order to increase hepatic gluconeogenesis in an attempt to meet the body's demands [8].

In diabetics, other causes of insufficient insulin include behavioral and technical etiologies. In some cases, diabetics may not administer the appropriate amount of insulin due to lack of compliance, whereas technical reasons include pump malfunctions. Behavioral reasons include inadequate insulin absorption secondary to lipohypertrophy from repeated injections at the same site instead of rotation to other areas on the body, clear of subcutaneous scarring.

Relative insulin deficiency may also occur when the concentrations of counter-regulatory hormones increase in response to stresses such as sepsis, trauma, and gastrointestinal illnesses. These conditions overwhelm homeostatic mechanisms and lead to metabolic decompensation despite taking the usual recommended dose of insulin [4]. It is critical that during these times, diabetics are properly instructed to increase their total daily dose of insulin in order to prevent hyperglycemia and/or ketogenesis.

Hyperglycemia

In DKA, hyperglycemia can initially develop for a number of reasons including iatrogenic, patient noncompliance, misguided glucose metabolism (persistent anabolic glucose production despite concurrent hyperglycemia/ euglycemia), and a surge of counter-regulatory hormones during stress as previously mentioned. Several medications have also been known to precipitate hyperglycemia by impairing insulin secretion/synthesis, increasing insulin resistance, and altering hepatic glucose metabolism such as steroids, immunosuppressants, high-dose thiazides, vasopressors, chemo-therapeutics and antipsychotics [9-11]. Furthermore, administration of IV fluids with dextrose in the absence of sufficient insulin will also lead to hyperglycemia.

Table 4. Medications associated with hyperglycemia [9-11]

Category	Drugs	Mechanism
Systemic Glucocorticoid	Prednisone, methylprednisolone, prednisolone, dexamethasone	Increased hepatic glucose production, increased insulin resistance, increased expression of peroxisome proliferator activated gamma receptors (PPAR-gamma)
Growth Hormone	Somatropin, tesamorelin	Increased counter-regulatory responses.
Immunosuppressants	Cyclosporine (ciclosporin), sirolimus, tacrolimus	Decreased insulin synthesis and release.
HIV Antiretrovirals	Protease Inhibitors nucleoside reverse transcriptase inhibitors (NRTIs)	Increased peripheral insulin resistance
Fluoroquinolones	Moxifloxacin	Altered insulin secretion
1st Generation Antipsychotics	Chlorpromazine, perphenazine, other phenothiazines	Appears to involve increased insulin resistance and diminished insulin secretion (not completely known)
2nd Generation Antipsychotics	Clozapine, iloperidone, olanzapine, paliperidone, quetiapine, risperidone	Appears to involve increased insulin resistance and diminished insulin secretion (not completely known)
Beta-Blockers	Atenolol, metoprolol, propranolol	Decreased insulin sensitivity
Lipid-altering	Niacin	Altered hepatic glucose metabolism
Thiazide diuretics	Hydrochlorothiazide, chlorthalidone, chlorothiazide, indapamide	Reduced total-body potassium, decreased insulin secretion and increased insulin resistance (usually associated with high-dose)
Vasopressors	Epinephrine, norepinephrine	Activation of glycogenolysis, increased hepatic gluconeogenesis, stimulation of glucagon and cortisol, inhibition of insulin secretion
Oral Contraceptives	Combination estrogen-progestogen oral contraceptives (> 35 mcg ethinyl estradiol), progestin only contraceptives	Altered hepatic glucose metabolism, increased peripheral insulin resistance.

Patient compliance plays a crucial role in appropriate glycemic control. Hyperglycemia occurs with excessive consumption of carbohydrate and sugar-containing beverages without appropriate insulin coverage. This is an especially prevailing issue with the increasing prevalence of obesity, partially due to poor nutritional options and poor knowledge of healthy dietary choices.

REPERCUSSIONS

With the body in an overall state of metabolic imbalance, during which hyperglycemia and inadequate insulin leading to impaired glucose utilization, the body experiences a number of characteristic repercussions as a result of this imbalance.

Ketone Production and Metabolic Acidosis

In DKA, metabolism inappropriately transitions into a fasting state resulting in a shift to catabolic processes. This includes lipolysis due to the combined effects of insulin deficiency and counter-regulatory hormone on hormone-sensitive lipase of adipocytes [6]. In this pathway, lipase releases fatty acids and glycerol from adipose tissue through lipolysis. Fatty acids are then linked to coenzyme A in the hepatocyte cytoplasm to form acyl-CoA, which is subsequently beta-oxidized to acetyl-CoA in the mitochondria. In the hormonal milieu of low insulin and high glucagon, this process is accelerated and leads to an accumulation of acetyl-CoA. A portion of the acetyl-CoA enters the Kreb cycle to produce ATP, while the excess acetyl-CoA is converted to acetoacetic acid. This acid may then be reduced to beta-hydroxybutyric acid or decarboxylated to acetone (chemically neutral).

Eventually, the acetoacetic acid and beta-hydroxybutyric acid (75% of circulating ketones) accumulate and decrease the body's pH leading to an anion gap metabolic acidosis [13, 14]. The overall severity is dependent on the rate and duration of ketone production, rate of excretion (dependent on renal function), adequacy of compensatory respiratory alkalosis, and the volume of distribution.

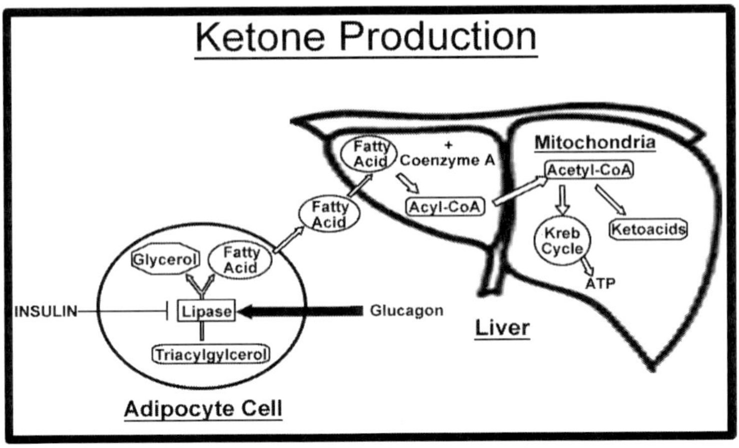

Figure 1. Lipolysis and ketone production [12].

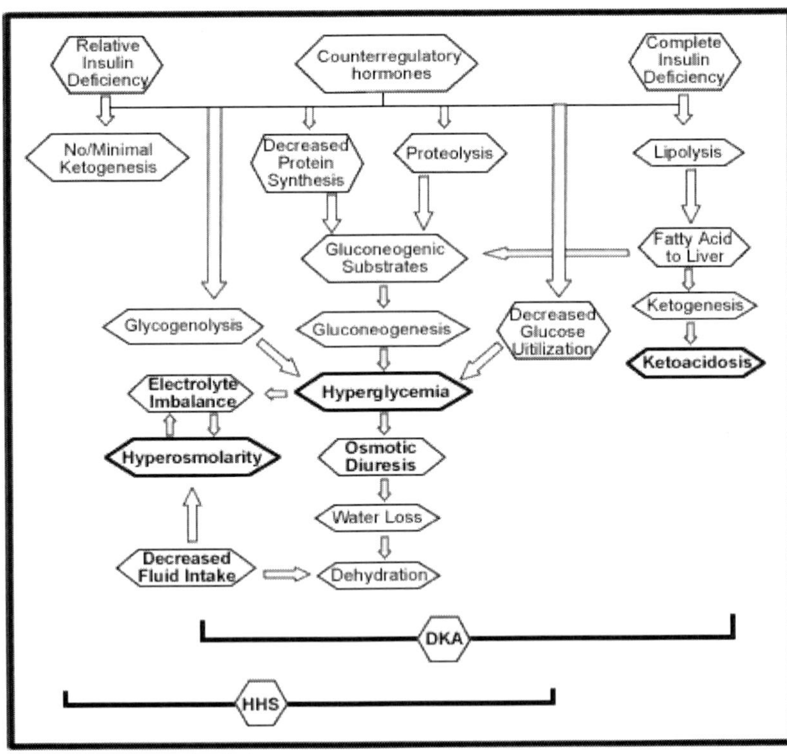

Figure 2. Pathogenesis of Diabetic Ketoacidosis and Hyperglycemic Hyperosmolar state [16].

DKA is a metabolic derangement characterized by a state of hyperglycemia, hyperosmolarity, and significant ketogenesis leading to acidosis. In addition, an alternative form of this metabolic derangement also occurs, known as a Hyperglycemic Hyperosmolar State (HHS), which is not characterized by the same degree of ketogensis. It occurs in diabetics with some endogenous insulin production (i.e., type 2 diabetics), which sufficiently suppresses ketosis but does not decrease hepatic gluconeogenesis. It is similarly associated with higher average levels of blood glucose (> 600 mg/dl) and higher osmolality (> 330 mOsm/kg); however, the pH is typically higher (> 7.25) and ketones are absent to mild. Though overall, the rate of hospital admissions for HHS is lower than for DKA and accounts for less than 1% of diabetic admissions, it is important to recognize and differentiate this state from DKA. HHS is characterized by more severe dehydration and fluid/electrolyte imbalances requiring a different management and can lead to significant morbidity and mortality if not adequately treated [15].

This state was previously seen almost exclusively in adults. However, with the growing number of children and adolescents with type 2 DM due to the rise in childhood obesity, it is becoming more common in the pediatric population. Most commonly, HHS, with and without DKA, is seen in undiagnosed adolescent African-American patients [17].

Dehydration and Electrolyte Imbalance

The hyperglycemia and acidemia of DKA are the primary causes of the associated electrolyte disturbances.

Glucose

Since glucose is restricted to the extracellular space in DKA, an increase in its concentration leads to an extracellular hyperosmolality osmotic pull of water out of cells causing dilution of extracellular solutes [18]. The hyperglycemia eventually leads to glucosuria, when the glucose level exceeds the renal threshold for glucose reabsorption (above 180 mg/dL). In turn, glucosuria creates an osmotic shift, leading to diuresis of free water, sodium and potassium. However, the concentration of electrolytes in the urine is much lower than that in the blood. This hyperosmolar state and subsequent diuresis can lead to dehydration. This is especially an issue for those who may have problems accessing and replenishing the free water losses such as young children, those with mental disabilities, and those who also have additional gastrointestinal sources of loss (e.g., vomiting).

Sodium

Hyperglycemia can have a marked effect on the body's sodium level. Dependent on the extent of the hyperglycemia, diuresis and fluid intake, a striking decrease in the concentration of sodium may manifest as the hyperglycemia-induced hyperosmolality shifts intracellular water in the extracellular space thus diluting the concentration of sodium and causing relative hyponatremia.

Potassium

In DKA, the potassium can be elevated, normal, or low. Both renal and gastrointestinal losses can result in an overall net loss of potassium. This and the hyperosmolar osmotic pull of intravascular water can lead to hypokalemia. Hypokalemia at presentation may be related to prolonged duration of DKA. Given that insulin permits the entry of potassium into the cell, its deficit typically presents with falsely high serum potassium. Hyperkalemia may also represent impaired renal function. With this in mind, health care providers must be reminded that with insulin administration, the net intracellular influx of potassium could lead to a significant hypokalemia without appropriate co-administration of potassium-containing fluids. In some cases, both of these processes occur concurrently and lead to an overall concentration that is within normal limits [3].

Phosphate

Generally, there is net negative phosphate balance due to decreased intake and phosphaturia caused by the osmotic diuresis. Despite this depletion, the level may be high or normal at initial presentation, due to extracellular shift of phosphate out of the cells in the presence of insulin deficiency and metabolic acidosis [19].

CONCLUSION

DKA remains a serious condition that is becoming more prevalent every year. Although it is both preventable and treatable, it is still a major cause of morbidity and mortality in the pediatric diabetic population. The best way to prevent DKA is to identify it early and anticipate the sequalae that might develop. It is therefore important for health care providers to recognize present-day risk factors that place patients at increased risk of developing DKA and to have ready access to appropriate resources to treat the anticipated complications.

REFERENCES

[1] Usher-Smith JA, Thompson MJ, Sharp SJ, Walter FM. Factors associated with the presence of diabetic ketoacidosis at diagnosis of diabetes in children and young adults: a systematic review. *BMJ* 2011; 343:d4092.
[2] Rewers A, Klingensmith G, Davis C, et al. Presence of diabetic ketoacidosis at diagnosis of diabetes mellitus in youth: the Search for Diabetes in Youth Study. *Pediatrics* 2008; 121:e1258.
[3] Dunger DB, Sperling MA, Acerini CL, et al. European Society for Paediatric Endocrinology/Lawson Wilkins Pediatric Endocrine Society consensus statement on diabetic ketoacidosis in children and adolescents. *Pediatrics* 2004; 113:e133.
[4] Wolfsdorf JI, Allgrove J, Craig ME, et al. Diabetic Ketoacidosis and hyperglycemic hyperosmolar state. *Pediatr Diabetes* 2014.; 15 Suppl 20:154.
[5] Rewers A, Chase HP, Mackenzie T, et al. Predictors of acute complications in children with type 1 diabetes. *JAMA* 2002; 287:2511.
[6] Foster DW. Banting lecture 1984. From glycogen to ketones--and back. *Diabetes* 1984; 33:1188.
[7] Cryer PE. Mechanisms of sympathoadrenal failure and hypoglycemia in diabetes. *J Clin Invest* 2006; 116:1470.
[8] Unger RH, Orci L. Glucagon and the A cell: physiology and pathophysiology (first two parts). *N Engl J Med* 1981; 304:1518.
[9] Sarafidis PA, Bakris GL. Antihypertensive treatment with beta-blockers and the spectrum of glycaemic control. *Q J Med* 2006; 99:431.
[10] Luna B, Feinglos MN. Drug-induced hyperglycemia. *JAMA* 2001; 286:1945.
[11] Thomas Z, Bandali F, McCowen K, et al. Drug induced endocrine disorders in the intensive care unit. *Crit Care Med* 2010; 38:S219.
[12] "New Diabetes March 2008." *New Diabetes March 2008*. N.p., n.d. Web. 02 Dec. 2014.

[13] Wolfsdorf JI. The International Society of Pediatric and Adolescent Diabetes guidelines for management of diabetic ketoacidosis: do the guidelines need to be modified? *Pediatr Diabetes* 2014; 15:277.

[14] Owen OE, Trapp VE, Skutches CL, et al. Acetone metabolism during diabetic ketoacidosis. *Diabetes* 1982; 31:242.

[15] Patel, Payal. "HHS vs DKA." *Endorama.* Chicago. 30 Oct. 2014. Lecture.

[16] "Pathogenesis DKA and HHS." *Diabetes Care* 29.12 (2006): n. pag. *Pathogenesis DKA and HHS*. American Diabetes Association. Web. 08 Dec. 2014.

[17] Fourtner SH, Weinzimer SA, Levitt Katz LE. Hyperglycemic hyperosmolar non-ketotic syndrome in children with type 2 diabetes. *Pediatr Diabetes* 2005; 6:129.

[18] Katz MA. Hyperglycemia-induced hyponatremia--calculation of expected serum sodium depression. *N Engl J Med* 1973; 289:843.

[19] Kebler R, McDonald FD, Cadnapaphornchai P. Dynamic changes in serum phosphorus levels in diabetic ketoacidosis. *Am J Med* 1985; 79:571.

In: Pediatric Diabetic Ketoacidosis ISBN: 978-1-63483-220-5
Editors: S. C. Duck and J. R. Hageman

Chapter 2

DIABETIC KETOACIDOSIS IN INFANTS AND YOUNG CHILDREN

Carmen D. Mironovici, MD, David Carmody, MD, and Siri Atma W. Greeley*, MD, PhD

Section of Pediatric and Adolescent Endocrinology
Comer Children's Hospital, Chicago, IL, US

ABSTRACT

Despite decades of advancements in technology to support the management of type 1 diabetes mellitus (T1DM), the disease requires intensive management and continues to be associated with significant morbidity. Diabetic ketoacidosis (DKA) is one of the most common and serious clinical complications of T1DM and is not only often present at diagnosis of diabetes, but can also be a recurrent problem in patients with suboptimal glycemic control long after diabetes diagnosis. The incidence of type 1 diabetes has been steadily increasing, with the greatest number of new cases occurring in children younger than five years of age. Since classic symptoms of diabetes are difficult to recognize in this younger age group, DKA is more often present at diagnosis. Furthermore, the youngest patients have a greater risk of other sequelae of DKA such as cerebral edema, even when the appropriate interventions are put in place. The diagnosis and management of DKA in early childhood therefore present unique challenges and differs significantly from older children

* Email: sgreeley@uchicago.edu.

and adults. Here we review clinical and therapeutic differences in this vulnerable group of patients.

INTRODUCTION

Type 1 diabetes mellitus (T1DM) is the most common metabolic disease of childhood, characterized by the inability to produce sufficient insulin due to chronic cellular-mediated autoimmune destruction of the beta cells in the pancreas. The prevalence of T1DM in children and adolescents is approximately 1 in 400-600, occurring most often in younger children, with a peak onset incidence around 11-13 years; this coincides with the timing of puberty, which may reflect the influence of a physiologic increase in insulin resistance. Less often, T1DM can occur in young adults or children as young as a year of age, although incidence among younger children appears to be increasing. A 2011 report from the United States (US) Centers for Disease Control and Prevention (CDC) estimated that, among children younger than 10 years of age, the annual rate of new cases was 19.7 per 100,000 population; among those 10 years or older, the rate was 18.6 per 100,000 population. Each year in the US, T1DM is newly diagnosed in 15,600 young people and is most common among non-Hispanic whites, followed by African Americans and Hispanic Americans. More males than females are affected; however, the incidence of diabetes does not differ by gender in those under the age of five [1].

There is strong evidence that incidence of T1DM in children has increased over the past few decades [2]. This increase appears largely confined to those aged under five years, with an annual increase varying from 3.5% [3] and 11% in more recent studies [1], with the most notable increase in children younger than 2 years of age. Interestingly, the incidence has remained low in children under 1 year of age. The EURODIAB Study, a large European survey for the period 1989-1998, showed similar annual increase in T1DM incidence (4.9%) among the 1 to 4 year age-group [4, 5]. Diabetes is no longer uncommon in toddlers and pre-school-aged children. This alarming trend towards younger age of onset reveals the increasing need for expert pediatric diabetes care.

ETIOLOGY

T1DM develops in genetically susceptible individuals as a result of progressive autoimmune destruction of beta cells in which environmental factors are believed to be involved as triggers, modifiers and promoters of this process [6-10]. Differences in autoimmune and genetic characteristics at presentation, and during the early course of clinical T1DM, suggest heterogeneity in the etiology and pathogenesis among children compared to adults. HLA haplotypes associated with disease susceptibility are more frequent in patients diagnosed during childhood than in those diagnosed during early adulthood. The rate of immunologically mediated beta-cell destruction appears to be more rapid in infants and children, with faster progression to complete loss of endogenous insulin production even after the clinical manifestation of T1DM [6]. As beta-cell mass declines, insulin secretion decreases until it becomes inadequate to maintain normal blood glucose levels. Very young children with T1DM are more likely to have a relative with T1DM, a higher prevalence of HLA susceptibility alleles, autoantibodies to pancreatic islet antigens at diagnosis, as well as a more rapid progression to failure of beta cells. The seasonal pattern of onset typical of older children is absent in those diagnosed under the age of five [1].

Polymorphisms of the class II human leukocyte antigen (HLA) genes that encode DR and DQ are the major genetic determinants of T1DM. Some studies have shown as many as 95% of patients with T1DM have either HLA-DR3 or HLA-DR4 and compound heterozygotes for both haplotypes are at significantly greater risk for T1DM than homozygotes. HLA-DQs (e.g., DQB1*02/*0302) are also considered specific, high risk markers of T1DM susceptibility, while other haplotypes are protective. Children diagnosed before the age of 2 years carry high-risk genotypes more often than older children. In one study, younger children with T1DM were less likely to carry the DQB1z/z protective genotype: only 17.2% of children under two, 20.3% of those aged 2.0-4.9 years, and 26.5% of children at or over 5 years old [6].

Given the genetic linkage to HLA, it is not surprising that most research points to T-cell dependent autoimmunity as the central cause of T1DM, with the humoral and innate arms of the immune system also appearing to play key roles. Although the strong association with HLA and high concordance among monozygotic twins point to the importance of genetic predisposition, unknown environmental factors strongly influence the likelihood of the autoimmune progression to disease in those at greatest genetic risk. For example, several lines of evidence have suggested that the targeting and/or progression of the autoimmune attack may be influenced by infections with enteroviruses, mumps, rubella and coxsackievirus B4; however direct evidence is lacking. For example, a nationwide, population-based cohort study in Taiwan demonstrated an association between enterovirus infection and the development of T1DM in children [11]. The concept that viral infections directly "cause" T1DM appears to be unlikely and rather viruses may represent one of several possible environmental factors that can potentially influence the course of the disease in genetically susceptible individuals.

Significant differences in autoantibody frequency and titers exist among patients manifesting T1DM at various ages [6, 12]. In one study, all children under 2 years of age tested positive for at least one of the diabetes-related antibodies at the time of diagnosis [13], with the very youngest children having the highest titers of insulin autoantibodies (IAA) and islet cell autoantibodies (ICA), whereas their titers of glutamic acid decarboxylase antibodies (GADA) were of the same magnitude to those in older children, and the titers of insulinoma-associated protein 2 (IA-2/ICA512) were lower than those of older children [14]. The proportion of children testing positive for all four antibodies was 53.1% in the youngest age-group, 42.0% in children 2-4.9 years and 26.9% in the oldest age-group ($p < 0.001$)[6]. While ICA is not considered useful in clinical practice, IAA, GAD and IA2 are commonly used to confirm the diagnosis of T1DM (as opposed to other types of diabetes such as monogenic forms), as is a newer test for zinc transporter 8 (ZnT8) autoantibodies.

Compared with older children, serum C-peptide levels are lower in 2-4 year old children at diagnosis and during follow-up [6]. Children diagnosed before 2 years of age have the lowest levels at diagnosis, suggesting poorly preserved residual beta-cell function. Furthermore, endogenous insulin secretion does not appear to recover after treatment of diabetes, whereas a substantial increase in serum C-peptide concentrations often occurs over the first 3 months following diagnosis in older age-groups. Accordingly, none of the children diagnosed before the age 2 years were in partial remission by the 6-month follow-up visit; however, 27.4% of the children aged 2.0-4.9 years and 37.1% of those diagnosed between 5.0 and 14.9 years of age were ($p < 0.001$).

Severity of DKA among the Very Young

Diabetic ketoacidosis (DKA) is a life-threatening metabolic derangement characterized by the triad of hyperglycemia, acidosis and ketonuria; DKA occurs rapidly in the absence of insulin. Younger age is associated with a higher frequency of DKA at diagnosis, as well as with more severe metabolic decompensation [6]. Even with appropriate intervention, DKA is associated with significant morbidity and mortality in the very young age group.

The current criteria for diagnosis of DKA published by the International Society for Paediatric and Adolescent Diabetes are: blood glucose > 11 mmol/L (> 200 mg/dL), venous pH < 7.30 or bicarbonate < 15 mmol/L and ketonemia and ketonuria. Its severity is defined by the degree of acidosis: mild, venous pH 7.2-7.3; moderate, pH 7.1-7.2; and severe if pH < 7.1 [15]. Progressive dehydration, hyperosmolarity, acidosis, and electrolyte disturbances exaggerate production of stress hormones that further promote a self-perpetuating cycle of progressive metabolic decompensation [6].

In several studies, more than half of children younger than 2 years of age presented with DKA as the first manifestation of T1DM [16, 17]. In addition, severe DKA (pH < 7.1) was seen in 10.0% of those younger than 2 years of age, but only in 2.9% of the patients in the group 2.0-4.9 years of age and in 4.7% of the patients in the group 5.0-14.9 years of age [6]. The severe metabolic decompensation seen in infants and young children may in part reflect a relatively greater loss of functional beta cell mass, given that children younger than 2 years of age have lower serum C-peptide concentrations at the diagnosis of diabetes [18] and also appear to lose their endogenous insulin secretory capacity faster than older children [17, 19].

It is unclear why some children present in DKA whereas others do not and whether the development of DKA is a consequence of delayed diagnosis, treatment or whether it reflects a particularly aggressive form of diabetes [20, 21]. Komulainen, et al.,. followed a group of probands having DKA at the diagnosis of T1DM and compared those with newly diagnosed T1DM patients who did not present in DKA [18]. In the ketoacidosis group, they observed low serum C-peptide concentrations, higher requirement of exogenous insulin, lower prevalence of remission, and worse diabetes control, as reflected by high glycated haemoglobin (HbA1c) concentrations. Their data clearly showed worse residual beta cell function in children with DKA at the diagnosis of the disease. The mean serum C-peptide concentration in the non-ketoacidosis group was significantly higher at the time of diagnosis and during the whole follow-up period than in the ketoacidosis group, even after adjustment for age and sex. A serum C-peptide concentration of 0.1 nmol/L or more was associated with favorable metabolic control. These differences were preserved for the whole 2 year observation period. The recommended amount of insulin was higher and partial remission was less common in the ketoacidosis than in the non-ketoacidosis group after adjustment for age. In spite of a larger dose of exogenous insulin, the ketoacidosis group had poorer glycemic control. The remission was considered to be a result of the functional recovery of the existing beta cells, which protected the child from developing DKA at diagnosis, and increasing peripheral insulin sensitivity after the initiation of insulin therapy. Similarly, children in the youngest age-group had higher HbA1c levels, reflecting the poorest metabolic control of this age-group [22].

FREQUENCY OF DKA, PRECIPITATING FACTORS AND PREVENTION STRATEGIES

In the US, the overall rates of DKA at the time of diagnosis have remained fairly constant at approximately 25% [16]. Children younger than 2 years and those older than 10 years are more susceptible to DKA than children between 2 and 10 years of age (< 2 y: 53%; 2-10 years: 16.9%; > 10 years: 33.3%) [18]. However, some studies suggest that the frequency of DKA at T1DM diagnosis may be decreasing among children younger than 5 years of age. In the Boston area, 43.7% of children diagnosed under 6 years of age had DKA at T1DM diagnosis during the 1990s [23] whereas a recent study reported a DKA frequency of 37.3% of children younger than 5 years of age [24]. These encouraging results indicate that more information and greater awareness may have led to earlier diagnosis with milder metabolic decompensation in these very young children. Education about the precipitating factors of DKA, a preventable complication of T1DM, and rapid access to health care providers contribute to better outcomes and fewer recurrences.

A meta-analysis including 46 studies involving more than 24 000 children in 31 countries [20] found that younger and poorer children are disproportionately affected by DKA at the time of their diagnosis of diabetes: children younger than 5 years of age, those from ethnic minority groups, lower family income, and lower parental educational achievement were at highest risk of DKA at T1DM diagnosis. Children were also more likely to later present in DKA if medical care was received but the signs and symptoms were attributed to a diagnosis other than diabetes ("diagnostic error"). Lack of health insurance (in the US) was also strongly associated with higher rates as well as greater severity of DKA at diagnosis; this may be related to a delay in seeking treatment, which was also associated with an increased risk of DKA. Lower body mass index (BMI) was associated with greater likelihood of DKA, which may reflect the association of obesity to type 2 diabetes and a lower risk of DKA. A preceding infection also increased risk of DKA, which could reflect a precipitating immune event or lead to a delay in diagnosis due to clinical error. In contrast, children with a first degree relative with T1DM, with parents with higher level of education, or who lived in an area with a higher background incidence of T1DM were less likely to present in DKA.

Table 1. Risk factors for DKA at original diagnosis of diabetes in children (adapted from reference 20)

Factors Increasing risk	Factors decreasing risk
Younger age	Family history of type 1 diabetes
Diagnostic error	Higher parental education
Ethnic minority status	Higher background incidence of type 1 diabetes
Lack of health insurance (in the US)	Presence of structured diabetes team
Lower body mass index	
Preceding infection	
Delayed treatment	
Lower socioeconomic status	
Unemployed mother	

Note: Factors are listed from top to bottom in decreasing order of strength of evidence, with those having been confirmed in the greatest number of studies being listed first.

Patient factors:

1. Age

Numerous studies showed that children younger than 2 years of age had three times the risk of presenting in DKA as children aged 2 years and older, and this association continued up to age 5. Several factors may explain the higher risk for DKA in younger children, including the frequent absence of classic symptoms of DKA, confusion with other intercurrent illnesses, and a shorter pre-clinical phase.

2. *Sex*

   One study reported a small but statistically significant increase in frequency in girls [25], whereas most other studies have not found any association to gender.
3. *Ethnicity*

   Despite T1DM and DKA being more common in white children in the US, several studies have found a consistently higher risk of DKA in African-american and non-white Hispanic minority groups compared to non-Hispanic white people [26].
4. *Insulin pump therapy*

   Some studies have shown an increase in risk for DKA in known diabetes patients treated with insulin pump therapy. This may be because only rapid- or short-acting insulin is used in pumps, so interruption of insulin delivery for any reason may rapidly leads to DKA unless treated appropriately. It is not clear how age might influence this risk and other studies have suggested that insulin pump therapy may be an especially good choice for younger children.
5. *BMI*

   There is a higher frequency of DKA in children with a lower BMI, which may reflect the lower likelihood of DKA in type 2 diabetes, which is strongly associated with obesity.
6. *Health insurance status*

   Several US studies reported that lack of private insurance was a risk factor for presenting in DKA, with significantly more patients with either Medicaid or no insurance presenting in DKA. Children with no insurance also had a greater risk of presenting in DKA compared with those receiving Medicaid.
7. *Household income*

   Lower household income has been associated with higher frequency of DKA [26].
8. *Preceding infection*

   A history of prior infection was the only disease-related factor associated with an increased risk of DKA. Infection is known to cause inflammation, pro-inflammatory cytokine release, and a counter regulatory response that collectively increase insulin resistance; if the increased requirements for insulin are not met, ketosis may ensue. The infection itself may also trigger more rapid autoimmune destruction of the beta cells. Alternatively, the presence of infection may mask the early symptoms of diabetes and make the diagnosis more difficult.

Clinician factors:

1. Diagnostic error

Children in whom the diagnosis of diabetes was not made at the first medical consultation had a threefold increased risk of presenting in DKA. One study found that significantly more children who presented with DKA had one or more medical consultations in the week before diagnosis [27]. The younger the child, the more difficult it is to obtain the classical history of polyuria, polydipsia and polyphagia with weight loss, especially as the disease was previously considered rare at an early age. Increased urination can be missed in infants or toddlers who are not toilet trained. Because of non-specific symptoms, the diagnostic error was significantly more likely to occur in infants and toddlers with diabetes, presenting in DKA or not. Acute infections, seen in more than half of the youngest children at the presentation of T1DM, may also mask the diabetic symptoms and signs, thus delaying the diagnosis.

Clinician/Patient factor:

1. Delay in appropriate treatment

Delay in treatment can be due to a patient delay in seeking treatment, or can be due to delay in making the appropriate diagnosis. Without treatment, the longer duration of symptoms (recognized or not) would lead to more severe dehydration, acidosis, and potentially severe complications such as cerebral edema or stroke. Children presenting with DKA had symptoms for a mean of 2 weeks and up to a third of them had at least one medical consultation in the week before diagnosis.

Prevention of recurrent DKA in young children with an established diagnosis of T1DM should focus on ensuring there is access to sufficient insulin and making caregivers aware of the increased risk of DKA, coma, and death in young children particularly when associated with infections [28]. Home ketone monitoring should be a standard part of diabetes management in children, with recommendations to check for ketones whenever blood glucoses are persistently elevated or during times of any illness. Some illnesses, especially those associated with fever, can raise blood glucose levels because of higher levels of stress hormones promoting gluconeogenesis and insulin resistance [29]. Illness often increases ketone body production too, because of inadequate insulin levels. Although home urine ketone monitoring is cheaper and more readily available, home measurement of beta-hydroxy butyrate (BOHB) concentrations in the blood of children diagnosed with diabetes enables earlier identification and treatment of ketosis, when compared to urine ketone testing [29]. Blood BOHB monitoring may be especially useful in very young children or when urine specimens are difficult to obtain. Blood ketones measurements may also be valuable to prevent DKA in patients who use an insulin pump. Elevations in blood BOHB may precede elevations in urine ketones due to interrupted insulin delivery (e.g., catheter occlusion or dislodgement), which can rapidly lead to ketogenesis and ketosis as well as increased insulin needs associated with intercurrent infections [30]. Caretakers and older pediatric patients themselves should be aware of the possible dissociation between urine ketones and blood BOHB concentrations [29].

COMPLICATIONS OF DKA

Cerebral edema (CE) is one of the most feared complications of DKA and occurs in 0.3-1% of DKA in children [28], typically 4-12 hours after initiation of treatment (but can occur before treatment has begun or at any time during treatment) and accounts for 55-87% of all DKA deaths [31-32]. Young age, especially less than five years, carries an increased risk for the development of cerebral edema. While this may reflect the more rapid deterioration in this age group and greater delay in diagnosis because of non-specificity of symptoms, it may also be due to greater susceptibility of the younger brain to metabolic and vascular changes associated with DKA. Greater severity at presentation in younger children associated with less maturity of cerebral and autoregulatory systems predispose children to CE [33]. Once CE develops, death occurs in 20-25% of patients and significant morbidity, including permanent neurologic injury and pituitary insufficiency, occurs in a substantial percentage of survivors (15-26%) [34-36]. The initial and typical CNS response to DKA is vasogenic edema. Many mechanisms have been proposed, including cerebral hypoperfusion with subsequent increased cerebral blood flow [34], the generation of various inflammatory mediators [37], a rapid shift in extracellular and intracellular fluids resulting in changes in osmolality and disruption of cellular membrane ion transport. Elevated ketones levels may disrupt membrane structure by causing oxidative tissue damage through production of reactive oxygen species and by compromising free radical scavenging. There is evidence of direct effects of ketones on brain microvascular endothelium that may alter permeability of the blood-brain barrier and contribute to CE.

Ketones were detected in the brain more frequently in children with altered mental status (restlessness, irritability, increased drowsiness, mental confusion, deterioration in level of consciousness, seizures, urinary incontinence) during treatment. Other symptoms and signs indicative of impending or present cerebral edema are headache, inappropriate bradycardia, recurrent vomiting, rising blood pressure, decreased oxygen saturation or specific neurological signs (cranial nerve palsies, pupillary response). Children younger than 5 years of age, those newly diagnosed with T1DM, especially presenting symptoms for longer duration before diagnosis have the highest risk for development of cerebral edema. Other risk factors are severe acidosis, profound hypočapnea and severe dehydration, reflected by with low pCO2 and increased serum high urea nitrogen at presentation [28]. Although imaging can confirm the presence of CE, radiological evidence can be delayed compared to clinical evidence [32]. Because of this and because CE can progress rapidly to severe neurological outcome or death, clinical suspicion for CE should prompt consideration of treatment with hypertonic saline or mannitol, with imaging being considered only if the patient is stable.

Complications such as mucormycosis and rhabdomyolysis are less frequently seen but gastropareis, hypokalemia and iatrogenic hypoglycemia may develop in young children. Frequent blood glucose and electrolyte monitoring and low dose insulin therapy may reduce the risk gastroparesis and hypokalemia.

Management of DKA

Successful treatment of DKA requires restoration of circulatory volume, a steady reduction of hyperglycemia, correction of electrolyte imbalances, identification of comorbid precipitating events and potential complications. DKA is a medical emergency in patients of all ages but young children in particular should be managed by experienced medical and nursing staff. Frequent monitoring of the patients' glucose and electrolytes should be coupled with regular evaluations of both the neurological and cardiovascular status. Clinical deterioration due to dehydration and acidosis develop more quickly in young children as mechanisms for metabolic compensation are less developed [38, 39]. Other factors, such as problems in cooperation, variable food intake and physical activity and parental fears of hypoglycemia may contribute to poor metabolic control in very young T1DM children [6, 40]. Children with severe DKA and those who are at increased risk for cerebral edema require immediate treatment in an intensive pediatric care unit, where heart rate, respiratory rate, blood pressure and intake and output, blood glucose and blood gas electrolytes, urea, and hematocrit will be frequently monitored and patients will benefit from hourly or more frequent neurological observation [28].

The most important initial therapeutic intervention is fluid replacement, followed by insulin administration. Correction of hypovolemia will improve decreased tissue perfusion and renal function, restore the GFR and enhance the clearance of glucose and ketones from the blood, also increasing the excretion of organic acids and reversing any lactic acidosis. There is a shift of water from the intracellular fluid compartment to the extracellular fluid compartment (ECF) in DKA, which determines the high effective osmolality of ECF. Rapid fluid replacement with hypotonic fluids, compared with isotonic, is associated with greater rises in intracranial pressure and increased risk of CE. A less rapid fluid deficit correction with isotonic or near-isotonic solutions will help prevent CE but will still efficiently correct the acidosis [28]. Therefore, Initial fluid resuscitation should involve only modest small boluses if needed based on clinically significant dehydration or cardiovascular compromise, otherwise the total volume deficit should be spread out by replacement over 36-48 hours. The youngest patients tend to have a higher basal metabolic rate and larger surface area relative to total body mass, and thus require greater precision in delivering fluids and electrolytes, which should generally be calculated based on surface area rather than weight [33]. Central lines in children with DKA are more frequently associated with thrombosis and should be used to only when absolutely necessary [33].

Most children with T1DM are profoundly insulin deficient. Insulin administration will stimulate peripheral glucose uptake while suppressing hepatic glucose production, lipolysis and ketogenesis. Insulin administration is thus necessary and will ensure reduction in hyperglucagonemia, reversal of the catabolic state and normalize lipid and protein metabolism. Intravenous insulin is typically stared at a dose of 0.1 U/Kg hourly as a continuous infusion, which will achieve steady-state serum insulin concentrations of 50-200 microU/ mL within 60 minutes, adequate to offset the insulin resistance characteristic of DKA. However insulin-sensitive patients, especially young children and those with mild-moderate DKA, may require lower doses of insulin, provided acidosis continues to resolve. Because rapid correction of glucose levels and osmolality is associated with worse outcome, careful attention should be paid to limit the fall in glucose to no more than 50-75 mg/dL per hour whenever possible. A more rapid decrease often occurs following fluid resuscitation even before insulin is started. It is thus reasonable in younger children or in patients with very high glucose levels (> 800 mg /dL) and/or hyperosmolality (> 330 mOsm/L) to delay insulin administration until the rate of fall in glucose/osmolality is apparent. In children younger than 4 years of age plasma glucose levels may take longer to fall to 210-250 mg/dL, presumably due to higher levels of growth hormone.

Potassium is lost from the intracellular pool as a result of hypertonicity, insulin deficiency and buffering of hydrogen ions within the cell, leading to severe total-body potassium deficiency. During acidosis, intracellular potassium enters the extracellular compartment and is loss in urine and emesis. Once insulin is substituted, it promotes uptake of potassium by cells and the serum potassium concentration may decrease abruptly. In this case, insulin therapy should be delayed until concentration is corrected to > 3.5 mEq/L to avoid cardiac arrhythmias and respiratory muscle weakness. Close monitoring of potassium levels is thus essential. Depletion of intracellular phosphate occurs in DKA as a result of osmotic diuresis. After starting IV insulin infusion, plasma phosphate will re-enter cells and a fraction will be excreted in the urine, determining a rapid decrease in plasma concentrations.

There is little evidence to support the use of bicarbonate in the treatment of DKA and is not recommended in young children as it may precipitate or worsen CE. Exogenous insulin will induce the metabolism of keto-anions, resulting in the regeneration of bicarbonate (HCO3) and spontaneous correction of acidemia [29]. Bicarbonate therapy may cause paradoxical CNS acidosis and that rapid correction of acidosis caused by bicarbonate will result in hypokalemia and may contribute to serum hypertonicity. In addition, alkali therapy may increase hepatic ketone production, thus slowing the rate of recovery from the ketosis.

In addition to the acute complications, presentation with DKA is also associated with future complications. At least one DKA event within 12 months occurred in 9.4% of the diabetic children younger than 6 years of age who participated in the T1D Exchange Clinic Registry [27]. Avoiding the initial DKA may facilitate good metabolic control over the first years of manifest T1DM [18] and prevent recurrent DKA, in which the related complications including coma and death occur more often [29]. Upon resolution of DKA, providers should use the patients' inpatient stay as an opportunity to provide additional diabetes education and training. Infants and toddlers are entirely dependent on caregivers for insulin therapy, nutrition and glucose monitoring, thus ensuring caregivers have appropriate diabetes education and psychosocial supports can reduce the risk of future complications.

Predisposing factors for DKA and precipitating illness should be sought and treated. Delay in diagnosis is common in younger children without a known history of diabetes. Recurrent DKA is typically due to insulin omission or inadequate insulin therapy during intercurrent illnesses. There are readily accessible local and international guidelines but support from senior medical staff should be sought early in the management of DKA in young children.

Conclusion

Diabetes in early childhood has a considerably greater impact on children and their families than it does in later years. DKA in adults is rarely associated with the devastating neurological sequelae that can occur in very young children. Clinicians should have a high index of suspicion for diabetes among younger children, as the classic symptoms of diabetes may be subtle and difficult to distinguish from other acute illnesses at this age. Improving public and clinician awareness of the signs and symptoms of hyperglycemia through structured diabetes education programs may decrease the delays in presentation and diagnosis. It is also important to continue diabetes education for caregivers of children with established T1DM on the use of insulin during illness and recognition of dehydration and ketonemia. DKA in early childhood has unique challenges and differs significantly from older patients and we encourage providers to seek guidance from clinicians experienced in the management of DKA in this vulnerable population.

References

[1] Gardner SG, Bingley PJ, Sawtell PA, et al. Rising incidence of insulin dependent diabetes in children aged under 5 years in the Oxford region: time trend analysis. *BMJ* 315:713, 1997.

[2] SEARCH Study Group: SEARCH for Diabetes in Youth: a multicenter study of the prevalence, incidence and classification of diabetes mellitus in youth. *Control Clin Trials* 25:458-471, 2004.

[3] Vehik K, Hamman RF, Lezotte D, et al. Increasing incidence of type 1 diabetes in 0-to-17 year-old Colorado youth. *Diabetes Care* 30:503-509, 2007.

[4] Libman IM, LaPorte RE. Changing trends in epidemiology of type 1 diabetes throughout the world: how far have we come and where do we go from here. *Pediatr Diabetes* 6:119-121, 2005.

[5] Karvonen M, Pitkaniemi J, Tuomilehto J. The onset age of type 1 diabetes in Finnish children has become younger: the Finnish Childhood Diabetes Registry group. *Diabetes Care* 22:1066-1070, 1999.

[6] Komulainen J, Kulmala P, Savola K, et al. Clinical, autoimmune, and genetic characteristics of very young children with type 1 diabetes. *Diabetes Care* 22:1950-1955, 1999.

[7] Dahlquist G. Environmental risk factors in human type 1 diabetes – an epidemiological perspective. *Diabetes Metab Rev* 11:37-46, 1995.

[8] Akerblom HK, Knip M. Putative environmental factors in type 1 diabetes. *Diabetes Metab Rev* 14:31-67, 1998.

[9] Lernmark A. Type 1 diabetes. *Clin Chem* 45:1331-1338; 1999.

[10] Atkinson MA, Eisenbarth GS, Michels, AW. Type 1 diabetes. *Lancet, 383*(9911), 69–82, 2014.

[11] Lin HC, Wang CH, Tsai FJ, et al. Enterovirus infection is associated with an increased risk of childhood type 1 diabetes in Taiwan: a nationwide population-based cohort study. *Diabetologia* 58(1), 79–86, 2015.

[12] Vehik K, Beam CA, Mahon JL, et al. Development of Autoantibodies in the TrialNet Natural History Study. *Diabetes Care* 34:1897-1901, 2011.

[13] Bingley PJ, Bonifacio E, Shattock M, et al. Can islet cell antibodies predict IDDM in general population? *Diabetes Care* 16:45-50, 1993.

[14] Komulainen J, Knip M, Lounamaa R, et al., and the Childhood Diabetes in Finland Study Group. Poor Beta-cell Function After the Clinical Manifestation of Type 1 Diabetes in Children Initially positive for Islet Cell Specific Autoantibodies. *Diabetic Medicine* 14:532-537, 1997.

[15] Wolfsdorf JI, Allgrove J, Craig ME et al., Diabetic ketoacidosis and hyperglycemic hyperosmolar state. *Pediatric Diabetes,* 15(S20), 154–179, 2014.

[16] Hekkala A, Reunanen A, Koski M, et al., Age-related differences in the frequency of ketoacidosis at diagnosis of type 1 diabetes in children and adolescents. *Diabetes Care* 33:1500-1502, 2010.

[17] Pinkney JH, Bingley PJ, Sawtell PA, et al. Presentation and progress of childhood diabetes mellitus: a prospective population-based study. *Diabetologia* 37:70-74, 1994.

[18] Komulainen J, Lounamaa R, Knip M, et al. Ketoacidosis at the diagnosis of type 1 (insulin dependent) diabetes mellitus is related to poor residual beta cell function. *Archives of disease in Childhood* 75:410-415, 1996.

[19] Sochett E, Daneman D, Clarson C, et al. Factors affecting and patterns of residual insulin secretion during the first year of type 1 (insulin-dependent) diabetes mellitus in children. *Diabetologia* 30:453-9, 1987.

[20] Usher-Smith JA, Thompson MJ, Sharp SJ, et al. Factors associated with the presence of diabetic ketoacidosis at diagnosis of diabetes in children and young adults: a systematic review. *BMJ* 343:d4092, 2011.

[21] Neu A, Ehehalt S, Willasch A, et al. Varying clinical presentations at onset of type 1 diabetes mellitus in children – epidemiological evidence for different subtypes of the disease? *Pediatr Diabetes* 2:147-53, 2001.

[22] Karges B, Meissner T, Icks A, et al. Management of diabetes mellitus in infants. *Nat Rev Endocrinol* 8:201-211, 2012.

[23] Quinn M, Fleischman A, Rosner B, et al. Characteristics at diagnosis of type 1 diabetes in children younger than 6 years. *J Pediatr* 148: 366-371, 2006.

[24] Rewers A, Klingensmith G, Davis C, et al. Presence of diabetic ketoacidosis at diagnosis of diabetes mellitus in youth: the Search for Diabetes in Youth Study. *Pediatrics* 121:e1258-e1266, 2008.

[25] Neu A, Willasch A, Ehehalt S, et al. Ketoacidosis at onset of type 1 diabetes mellitus in children – frequency and clinical presentation. *Pediatr Diabetes* 4:77-81, 2003.

[26] Cengiz E, Dongyuan X, Wong JC, et al. Severe Hypoglycemia and Diabetic Ketoacidosis among Youth with Type 1 Diabetes in the T1D Exchange Clinic Registry. *Pediatr Diabetes* 14 (6):447-454, 2013.

[27] Bui H, To T, Stein R. et al. Is diabetic ketoacidosis at disease onset a result of missed diagnosis? *J Pediatr* 156:472-7, 2010.

[28] Dunger DB, Sperling MA, Acerini CL et al. ESPE/LWPES consensus statement on diabetic ketoacidosis in children and adolescents. *Arch Dis Child* 89:188-194, 2004.

[29] Brink S, Joel D, Laffel L et al. Sick day management in children and adolescents with diabetes. *Pediatric Diabetes* 15:193-202, 2014.

[30] Rayfield EJ, Ault MJ, Keusch GT, et al. Infections and diabetes : the case for glucose control. *Am J Med* 72:439-50, 1982.

[31] Rosenbloom AL. Intracerebral crises during treatment of diabetic ketoacidosis. *Diabetes Care* 13:22-33, 1990.

[32] Marcin JP, Glaser N, Barnett P, et al. Factors associated with adverse outcomes in children with diabetic ketoacidosis-related cerebral edema. *J Pediatr* 141:793-797, 2002.

[33] Wolfsdorf J, Glaser N, Sperling MA. Diabetic ketoacidosis in infants, children and adolescents: a consensus statement from the American Diabetes Association. *Diabetes Care* 29:1150-9, 2006.

[34] Glaser N, Barnett P, McCaslin I, et al. Risk factors for cerebral edema in children with diabetic ketoacidosis. The Pediatric Emergency medicine Collaborative Research Committee of the American Academy of Pediatrics. *N Engl J Med* 344:264-269, 2001.

[35] Edge JA, Hawkins MM, Winter DL, et al. The risk and outcome of cerebral oedema developing during diabetic ketoacidosis. *Arch Dis Child* 85:16-22, 2001.

[36] Lawrence SE, Cummings EA, Gaboury I, et al. Population-based study of incidence and risk factors for cerebral edema in pediatric diabetic ketoacidosis. *J pediatr* 146:688-692, 2005.

[37] Abbott NJ. Inflammatory mediators and modulation of blood-brain barrier permeability. *Cell Mol Neurobiol* 20:131-147, 2000.

[38] Salman H, Abanamy A, Ghassan B, et al. Insulin-dependent diabetes mellitus in children: familial and clinical patterns in Riyadh. *Ann Saudi Med* 11:302-6, 1991.

[39] Samuelsson U, Stenhammar L. Clinical characteristics at onset of type 1 diabetes in children diagnosed between 1977 and 2001 in the south-east region of Sweden. *Diabetes Res Clin Pract* 68:49-55, 2005.

[40] American Diabetes Association. Standards of medical care in diabetes – 2015. *Diabetes Care* 38 Suppl 1: S 5-85, 2015.

In: Pediatric Diabetic Ketoacidosis ISBN: 978-1-63483-220-5
Editors: S. C. Duck and J. R. Hageman

Chapter 3

KETOSIS-PRONE TYPE 2 DIABETES MELLITUS IN CHILDREN AND ADOLESCENTS

Orit Pinhas-Hamiel*, MD, and Philip Zeitler, MD, PhD
Pediatric Endocrinology and Diabetes, Edmond and Lily Safra Children's Hospital, Sheba Medical Center, Tel-Hashomer, Ramat-Gan, Sackler School of Medicine, Tel-Aviv University, Israel
Section of Endocrinology, Department of Pediatrics, University of Colorado School of Medicine, Aurora, CO, US

ABSTRACT

A subset of adolescents with T2DM appears to be at increased risk for development of Diabetic ketoacidosis (DKA) at the time of diagnosis. The highest prevalence of DKA at onset is observed in African-American adolescents, reaching up to 25%. DKA at onset of T2DM in youth has also been described in Japan, Thailand, and Canada. Adolescents with T2DM presenting with DKA are extremely obese, with markedly elevated HbA1c levels at presentation. Known precipitants for the episode of DKA are severe infections and exposure to atypical antipsychotic drugs, however, most often no specific etiology is identified. Acute complications, such as cerebral edema, have been described in adolescent with T2DM. The discrimination between T1DM

* Correspondence to: Dr Orit Pinhas-Hamiel, Pediatric Endocrinology and Diabetes, Edmond and Lily Safra Children's Hospital, Sheba Medical Center, Tel-Hashomer, Ramat-Gan, 52621, Israel. Tel 972-3-5305015; Fax 972-3-5305055.

and T2DM in an individual with new onset diabetes presenting with DKA is extremely difficult on clinical grounds alone.

INTRODUCTION

Diabetic ketoacidosis (DKA) is a life-threatening yet preventable condition and has been considered a hall mark of type 1 diabetes mellitus (T1DM). The characteristics of DKA are hyperglycemia, hyperketonemia and metabolic acidosis. DKA is defined as $pH < 7.35$ and $HCO_2 < 15$ mEq/l in the presence of hyperglycemia. Ketonuria is defined as urinary ketones > 15 mg/dl ("small"). A systematic review that assessed 65 cohorts in 31 countries reported that up to 80% of new onset T1DM presented in DKA [1]. However, accumulating evidence from both adults and adolescents diagnosed with type 2 diabetes mellitus (T2DM) has demonstrated that DKA is not limited to T1DM. The literature on DKA in youth-onset T2DM is limited, but we review here what is known about the prevalence of DKA in adolescents with new- onset T2DM, its precipitants, and outcomes.

PATHOPHYSIOLOGY

The occurrence of DKA, whether in T1DM or T2DM, is the result of insufficient insulin to fully suppress lipolysis. In T1DM, this is generally due to absolute insulin deficiency as a consequence of β-cell destruction. In T2DM, current data suggest that, in a subgroup of patients, ketoacidosis is caused by an acute reduction in insulin secretion and action on the background of severe insulin resistance [2]. Adult patients with ketosis-prone T2DM had impaired insulin response to oral and intravenous glucose and to arginine, as well as impaired glucagon suppression, suggesting that both β- and α-cell dysfunction contribute to the development of DKA [3]. Furthermore, lipolysis is particularly resistant to suppression in adolescents with T2DM, creating a situation in which even relative decreases in insulin secretion in these highly resistant individuals are sufficient to allow lipolysis to occur [4].

EPIDEMIOLOGY

Among Adults

Among adult patients, those who present with DKA but subsequently have clinical and metabolic features characteristic of T2DM have been classified as having atypical diabetes. This presentation is also called diabetes type 1B, idiopathic type 1 diabetes, atypical diabetes, Flatbush diabetes, type 1.5 diabetes, and more recently and most appropriately, ketosis-prone T2DM [5]. The prevalence of ketosis-prone T2DM is not known. It is most common in African-Americans and accounts for 25% to 50% of new-onset diabetes cases presenting with DKA. It has also been described in Hispanic, Native-American, Japanese, Chinese, Hispanic, and White populations [5].

Among Children and Adolescents

The first study reporting the occurrence of DKA in children with T2DM was from Cincinnati [6]. Twenty-five percent of obese African-American adolescents with negative islet cell antibodies presented with DKA and 42% with ketonuria. Since then several other case reports [7, 8], case series [9-11] and population-based studies [12] have been published. Table 1 summarizes the prevalence of DKA and ketonuria in several populations. Interestingly despite the high prevalence of T2DM among Pima Indians and individuals from Nauru, we could not find reports regarding DKA among these populations.

1. Two interesting lessons can be drawn from these data. 1. The highest prevalence of DKA is observed in African-American adolescents. Similarly ketonuria was most prevalent in African-American and African Canadian adolescents. This is in agreement with the increased prevalence of DKA among African-American adults with T2DM. The reasons for this greater prevalence of ketosis-prone T2DM among African-American adolescents is not clear, but studies have shown that, for the same degree of insulin sensitivity, insulin secretion is higher in African American children, possibly leading to earlier β-cell exhaustion in the setting of long-standing resistance and lower insulin secretion at presentation of diabetes, leading to greater risk for ketosis [13].

Table 1. Prevalence of DKA and ketonuria in children and adolescents with T2DM

Place	Age (years)	Ethnicity	n of patients with T2DM	% with Ketonuria	% with DKA	Year	Author
Cincinnati, Ohio	10-17	African American	28	42	25	1982-1995	Pinhas-Hamiel [6]
		White	12	0	0		
Winnipeg, Manitoba, Canada	6-18	Aboriginal origin	120	NA	4.2	1986-1999	Sellers [10]
Arkansas	8-19	74%AA, 24% whites 2% Hispanic	50	18	> 25	1988-1995	Scott [9]
Australia	< 19	53% of Indigenous origin	23		5	1990-2002	McMahon [28]
US Bronx NY	< 18	AA Caribbean-Hispanic	89	35	5.6	1990-2000	Grinstein [29]
Japan	< 20		36	30.5		1992-2001	Matsui [14]
Toronto, Canada	< 18	Overall	44	30	8	1994-2002	Zdravkovic [11]
		AA		45	18		
		Asian		21	5		
		Hispanic		25	0		
		Caucasians		33	0		
Thailand	12.1 ± 2.3		26		19.2	2005	Likitmaskul [30]
SEARCH	10-19				11.7	2002–2003	Dabelea [12]
SEARCH	< 20		507		9.7	2002-2004	Rewers [23]
SEARCH	10-19				6.3	2004–2005	Dabelea [12]
SEARCH	10-19				5.7	2008–2010	Dabelea [12]

2. Data from the SEARCH study, a population-based study in geographically defined populations in the states of Ohio, Washington, South Carolina, and Colorado; and among Indian Health Service beneficiaries in American Indian populations in Arizona and New Mexico; shows a significant ~ 10% per year decrease in the prevalence of DKA in adolescents. This finding may reflect earlier diagnosis or increased public awareness of the early symptoms of diabetes [12].

Characteristics of Adolescents Presenting with T2DM and DKA

Weight

Reflecting the obesity characteristic of adolescents diagnosed with T2DM, those presenting with DKA are extremely obese. For example, Valabhji et al., [8] reported DKA in 16 and 17-year old adolescents whose weights were 124 kg and 135 kg, with body mass index (BMI) of 46.1 kg /m^2 and 39.9 kg /m^2 respectively.

Metabolic Control

The common denominator in all studies reporting DKA in T2DM is poor glycemic control at the time of presentation, with markedly elevated HbA1c levels (mean HbA1c 13.9 ± 2.6%) [10] suggesting long-standing hyperglycemia.

Gender

Among adults, several series of patients with ketosis-prone T2DM show a 2-or 3-fold higher prevalence in men [5]. In Cincinnati, the sex distribution of adolescents with DKA reflected the sex distribution of the population with T2DM. In Canada, a female predominance was identified, whereas in the US the SEARCH study reported that males had significantly higher DKA prevalence [8]. Among Japanese with youth-onset T2DM, the male to female ratio for patients with ketonuria was remarkably high (10:1) [14] compared to the group without ketonuria. All together these data suggest variability in the gender distribution in different ethnic groups.

Age

DKA at onset of T2DM appears to be more common among youth aged 10 to 14 years than in 15- to19-year-old youth. Importantly, children younger than 10 years presenting with DKA and having T2DM have been reported (17 cases), including a case of a 7-year-old with new-onset T2DM presenting with severe DKA [7].

Precipitant Factors

Among subjects with T1DM, multiple factors affect the risk of developing DKA at onset. These include preceding infection, minority ethnicity, lack of health insurance, delayed treatment, and low BMI [15]. Other risk factors that have been identified to be inversely associated with DKA in T1DM are a country's gross domestic product, latitude, and background incidence of T1DM.

Similarly, among children and adolescents with T2DM, obvious precipitants for the episode of DKA were severe infections, such as sepsis, pneumonia, gonoccoccal septicemia [10] and osteomyelitis. However, in several studies only a minority of cases had acute illness [10]. As mentioned above, minority ethnicity is also a risk factor, whereas, the role of parental education, health insurance, or household income in youth with T2DM has not established due to small numbers [12]. In T1DM, having a first degree relative with T1DM is a protective factor for DKA. However, among adolescents with T2DM, a positive family history of T2DM was found in the majority of the subjects yet this did not lead to early recognition of symptoms.

Atypical antipsychotics are associated with increased risk of developing T2DM in adults and adolescents [16]. Although rare, exposure to atypical antipsychotic drugs has also been linked with increased risk of DKA in adolescents. A case of ketosis in a 7 year-old boy and acute DKA in a16-year-old girl during olanzapine therapy have been reported [17, 18.] The precise underlying mechanism of the metabolic side effects of atypical antipsychotics is not clear. Interestingly it appears that weight gain is not the only contributor. Although 84% of adults treated with atypical antipsychotics who developed T2DM or DKA were overweight before antipsychotic treatment, 50% manifested no weight gain [19]. Furthermore, even "weight neutral" antipsychotics, such as aripiprazole, have been linked to DKA [20]. Animal studies have confirmed acute derangements in glucose metabolism after only a single dose of atypical antipsychotics. Similarly, a single-dose of olanzapine in healthy volunteers resulted in raised fasting glucose over 4.25 hours [21]. As the prescription of antipsychotics has expanded dramatically in the last decade among children and adolescents, their adverse side effects on development of DKA should be considered.

Finally, excessive ingestion of sugar-containing soft drinks has been described among young Japanese presenting with DKA [22]. It is suggested that acute loss of insulin secretion due to glucotoxicity resulted from excessive consumption of these drinks.

Discriminating between T1DM and T2DM in New Onset Diabetes Presenting with DKA

The reports of DKA in T2DM, affecting all ages and ethnic groups [23], make it clear that discrimination between T1DM and T2DM in new onset diabetes presenting with DKA is extremely difficult. In these circumstances, it is important to consider markers of autoimmunity (GAD, IA2, insulin, and ZnT8 antibodies) and HLA genotype [24].

Course

Acute Course

Cerebral edema is a severe outcome of DKA occurring in about 1% of cases of children with T1DM. Although rare, cerebral edema is a life-threatening complication, 1-in-5 affected T1DM patients die, and up to one-third will have neurologic deficits and morbidity [25].

A case report of a 15- year- old African-American female diagnosed with T2DM and DKA who developed cerebral edema was reported. Interestingly she developed cerebral edema before initiation of therapy [26]. High physicians' index of suspicion contributed to this patient's full recovery. A case of a 7-year-old girl with new-onset diabetes reported as T2DM and presenting with severe DKA whose neurologic status deteriorated dramatically without cerebral edema has been documented [7]. There is also a published case of new-onset diabetes reported as T2DM presenting as DKA concomitant with pneumomediastinum and Mallory-Weiss tear in a young boy [27].

Long-term Course

Data from follow-up studies of adults with ketosis-prone T2DM show that 70% of patients have at least one repeat episode of acute hyperglycemia or DKA within two years if treated with diet and lifestyle changes alone. This risk for severe deterioration is likely a reflection of the lower insulin secretion in these individuals.

There are limited data on the long-term follow up of adolescents with T2DM who presented with DKA. Compared to lean children, half of obese children with DKA achieved near normoglycemia and discontinued insulin therapy within 2.2 ± 2.3 months of follow-up, while none of the lean children discontinued insulin therapy. Despite this initial favorable response, 78% of obese children who achieved remission ultimately relapsed into hyperglycemia and required insulin treatment (time to relapse: 19.2 ± 17 months) [24].

TREATMENT

Treatment of DKA in new-onset T2DM is the same as treatment in T1DM, though the degree of hyperglycemia and hyperosmolality may be greater. As in T1DM, acute treatment consists of intravenous fluids and intravenous insulin. The presence of precipitating factors should be considered, including infection and medications. In most cases subsequent to acute presentation, insulin doses can be gradually reduced as oral antihyperglycemic agents (generally metformin) are initiated and insulin therapy ultimately discontinued altogether. Near-normoglycemic remission is achieved in most cases on metformin alone.

CONCLUSION

A subset of adolescents with T2DM appears to be at increased risk for development of ketosis, including DKA, at the time of diagnosis and subsequently. Therefore, as T2DM becomes more prevalent, the prevalence of DKA in T2DM is also rising. The presence of DKA at diagnosis cannot be used to support the diagnosis of T1DM or, alternatively, as evidence against the diagnosis of T2DM. Extreme obesity and the use of atypical antipsychotics should increase suspicion. There is a need for increased awareness of the occurrence of DKA among adolescents with T2DM among health care providers.

REFERENCES

[1] Usher-Smith JA, Thompson M, Ercole A, Walter FM: Variation between countries in the frequency of diabetic ketoacidosis at first presentation of type 1 diabetes in children: A systematic review. *Diabetologia* 2012;55:2878-2894.

[2] Misra S, Oliver N, Dornhorst A: Diabetic ketoacidosis: Not always due to type 1 diabetes. *Bmj* 2013;346:f3501.

[3] Choukem SP, Sobngwi E, Fetita LS, Boudou P, De Kerviler E, Boirie Y, Hainault I, Vexiau P, Mauvais-Jarvis F, Calvo F, Gautier JF: Multitissue insulin resistance despite near-normoglycemic remission in africans with ketosis-prone diabetes. *Diabetes Care* 2008;31:2332-2337.

[4] Kelsey MM, Forster JE, Van Pelt RE, Reusch JE, Nadeau KJ: Adipose tissue insulin resistance in adolescents with and without type 2 diabetes. *Pediatr Obes* 2014;9:373-380.

[5] Umpierrez GE, Smiley D, Kitabchi AE: Narrative review: Ketosis-prone type 2 diabetes mellitus. *Ann Intern Med* 2006;144:350-357.

[6] Pinhas-Hamiel O, Dolan LM, Zeitler PS: Diabetic ketoacidosis among obese african-american adolescents with niddm. *Diabetes Care* 1997;20:484-486.

[7] Stephen MD, Gungor N, Douty DR: Type 2 diabetes mellitus in a young girl: Ominous presentation and atypical course. *J Pediatr Endocrinol Metab* 2012;25:577-580.

[8] Valabhji J, Watson M, Cox J, Poulter C, Elwig C, Elkeles RS: Type 2 diabetes presenting as diabetic ketoacidosis in adolescence. *Diabet Med* 2003;20:416-417.

[9] Scott CR, Smith JM, Cradock MM, Pihoker C: Characteristics of youth-onset noninsulin-dependent diabetes mellitus and insulin-dependent diabetes mellitus at diagnosis. *Pediatrics* 1997;100:84-91.

[10] Sellers EA, Dean HJ: Diabetic ketoacidosis: A complication of type 2 diabetes in canadian aboriginal youth. *Diabetes Care* 2000;23:1202-1204.

[11] Zdravkovic V, Daneman D, Hamilton J: Presentation and course of type 2 diabetes in youth in a large multi-ethnic city. *Diabet Med* 2004;21:1144-1148.

[12] Dabelea D, Rewers A, Stafford JM, Standiford DA, Lawrence JM, Saydah S, Imperatore G, D'Agostino RB, Jr., Mayer-Davis EJ, Pihoker C: Trends in the prevalence of ketoacidosis at diabetes diagnosis: The search for diabetes in youth study. *Pediatrics* 2014;133:e938-945.

[13] Weiss R, Dziura JD, Burgert TS, Taksali SE, Tamborlane WV, Caprio S: Ethnic differences in beta cell adaptation to insulin resistance in obese children and adolescents. *Diabetologia* 2006;49:571-579.

[14] Matsui J, Tamasawa N, Tanabe J, Kasai N, Murakami H, Matsuki K, Suda T: Clinical characteristics of japanese youth-onset type 2 diabetes with ketonuria. *Diabetes Res Clin Pract* 2005;70:235-238.

[15] Usher-Smith JA, Thompson MJ, Sharp SJ, Walter FM: Factors associated with the presence of diabetic ketoacidosis at diagnosis of diabetes in children and young adults: A systematic review. *Bmj* 2011;343:d4092.

[16] Bobo WV, Cooper WO, Stein CM, Olfson M, Graham D, Daugherty J, Fuchs DC, Ray WA: Antipsychotics and the risk of type 2 diabetes mellitus in children and youth. *JAMA Psychiatry* 2013;70:1067-1075.

[17] Courvoisie HE, Cooke DW, Riddle MA: Olanzapine-induced diabetes in a seven-year-old boy. *J Child Adolesc Psychopharmacol* 2004;14:612-616.

[18] Selva KA, Scott SM: Diabetic ketoacidosis associated with olanzapine in an adolescent patient. *J Pediatr* 2001;138:936-938.

[19] Jin H, Meyer JM, Jeste DV: Phenomenology of and risk factors for new-onset diabetes mellitus and diabetic ketoacidosis associated with atypical antipsychotics: An analysis of 45 published cases. *Ann Clin Psychiatry* 2002;14:59-64.

[20] Church CO, Stevens DL, Fugate SE: Diabetic ketoacidosis associated with aripiprazole. *Diabet Med* 2005;22:1440-1443.

[21] Hahn MK, Wolever TM, Arenovich T, Teo C, Giacca A, Powell V, Clarke L, Fletcher P, Cohn T, McIntyre RS, Gomes S, Chintoh A, Remington GJ: Acute effects of single-dose olanzapine on metabolic, endocrine, and inflammatory markers in healthy controls. *J Clin Psychopharmacol* 2013;33:740-746.

[22] Yamada K, Nonaka K: Diabetic ketoacidosis in young obese japanese men. *Diabetes Care* 1996;19:671.

[23] Rewers A, Klingensmith G, Davis C, Petitti DB, Pihoker C, Rodriguez B, Schwartz ID, Imperatore G, Williams D, Dolan LM, Dabelea D: Presence of diabetic ketoacidosis at diagnosis of diabetes mellitus in

youth: The search for diabetes in youth study. *Pediatrics* 2008;121:e1258-1266.

[24] Low JC, Felner EI, Muir AB, Brown M, Dorcelet M, Peng L, Umpierrez GE: Do obese children with diabetic ketoacidosis have type 1 or type 2 diabetes? *Prim Care Diabetes* 2012;6:61-65.

[25] Tasker RC, Acerini CL: Cerebral edema in children with diabetic ketoacidosis: Vasogenic rather than cellular? *Pediatr Diabetes* 2014;15:261-270.

[26] Morales AE, Daniels KA: Cerebral edema before onset of therapy in newly diagnosed type 2 diabetes. *Pediatr Diabetes* 2009;10:155-157.

[27] Lin SY, Chang CT, Chen CC, Wang TY: Diabetic ketoacidosis complicated by pneumomediastinum and mallory-weiss tear in a young boy with new onset type 2 diabetes. *South Med J* 2008;101:769-770.

[28] McMahon SK, Haynes A, Ratnam N, Grant MT, Carne CL, Jones TW, Davis EA: Increase in type 2 diabetes in children and adolescents in western australia. *Med J Aust* 2004;180:459-461.

[29] Grinstein G, Muzumdar R, Aponte L, Vuguin P, Saenger P, DiMartino-Nardi J: Presentation and 5-year follow-up of type 2 diabetes mellitus in african-american and caribbean-hispanic adolescents. *Horm Res* 2003;60:121-126.

[30] Likitmaskul S, Santiprabhob J, Sawathiparnich P, Numbenjapon N, Chaichanwatanakul K: Clinical pictures of type 2 diabetes in thai children and adolescents is highly related to features of metabolic syndrome. *J Med Assoc Thai* 2005;88 Suppl 8:S169-175.

In: Pediatric Diabetic Ketoacidosis ISBN: 978-1-63483-220-5
Editors: S. C. Duck and J. R. Hageman

Chapter 4

MANAGEMENT OF PEDIATRIC DIABETIC KETOACIDOSIS IN THE EMERGENCY DEPARTMENT

Michelle Lemelman[1,*], MD, Joseph R. Hageman[1,2], MD, Heather Fagan[3], MD, Lisa McQueen[1], MD, and Stephen C. Duck[2], MD

[1]Pediatric Endocrinology and Diabetes, Department of Pediatrics, Comer Children's Hospital, University of Chicago Medical Center, Chicago, Illinois, US

[2]Pediatric Endocrinology, Northshore University HealthSystem, Evanston, Illinois, US

[3]Nemours Children's Hospital, Orlando, Florida, US

ABSTRACT

Optimal management of pediatric patients with diabetic ketoacidosis (DKA) begins with prompt recognition of the diagnosis, followed by thoughtful initiation of therapy including isotonic fluid infusion for dehydration, replacement of insulin deficiency using intravenous insulin

* Correspondence to: Dr Michelle Blanco, University of Chicago Medical Center, Department of Pediatrics, 5721 South Maryland Avenue, MC8016 Chicago Illinois, 60637. Tel 773-702-6435, Fax: 773-834-0748, Michelle.blanco@uchospitals.edu. No financial disclosures for this manuscript.

infusion, and correction of electrolyte abnormalities. Hourly monitoring of vital signs and mental status as well as blood glucose levels are essential. Virtually all of these initial steps take place in the emergency department pending further disposition and transfer to an intensive care setting. We present data from a characterization of practice in emergency departments in the State of Illinois as an example of the variation in management and outline best practice management based on new guidelines published in the peer review literature by the pediatric endocrine societies. Prevention of cerebral edema and other serious sequelae in this group of patients with DKA is essential.

Introduction/Background

Diabetes mellitus is caused by a relative or total deficiency of insulin, normally produced by the pancreas. Approximately one third of patients with Type I diabetes mellitus present with diabetic ketoacidosis (DKA), characterized by hyperglycemia, metabolic acidosis with a low bicarbonate level and evidence of an accumulation of ketoacids in the blood [1]. With a decrease in effective circulating insulin, there is an increase in counter-regulatory hormones including catecholamines, cortisol, growth hormone and glucagon leading to increased gluconeogensis in the liver. With increases in glucose and little to no insulin to allow for glucose utilization, the patient is commonly left with hyperosmolarity and ketone body production.

In 2010, the Centers for Disease Control and Prevention estimated that 215,000 Americans younger than 20 years old had Type 1 diabetes. Frequency of DKA at disease onset is 15-67% in Europe and North America and 1 to 10% per patient per year in children with established Type I Diabetes Mellitus (TIDM) [2]. Severe complications of DKA in children include cerebral edema, permanent neurologic deficits, and long-term memory dysfunction. Although this illness is predominantly managed in pediatric intensive care units, these patients frequently present to, and are acutely managed in, emergency departments.

DKA Management in the Pediatric Emergency Department

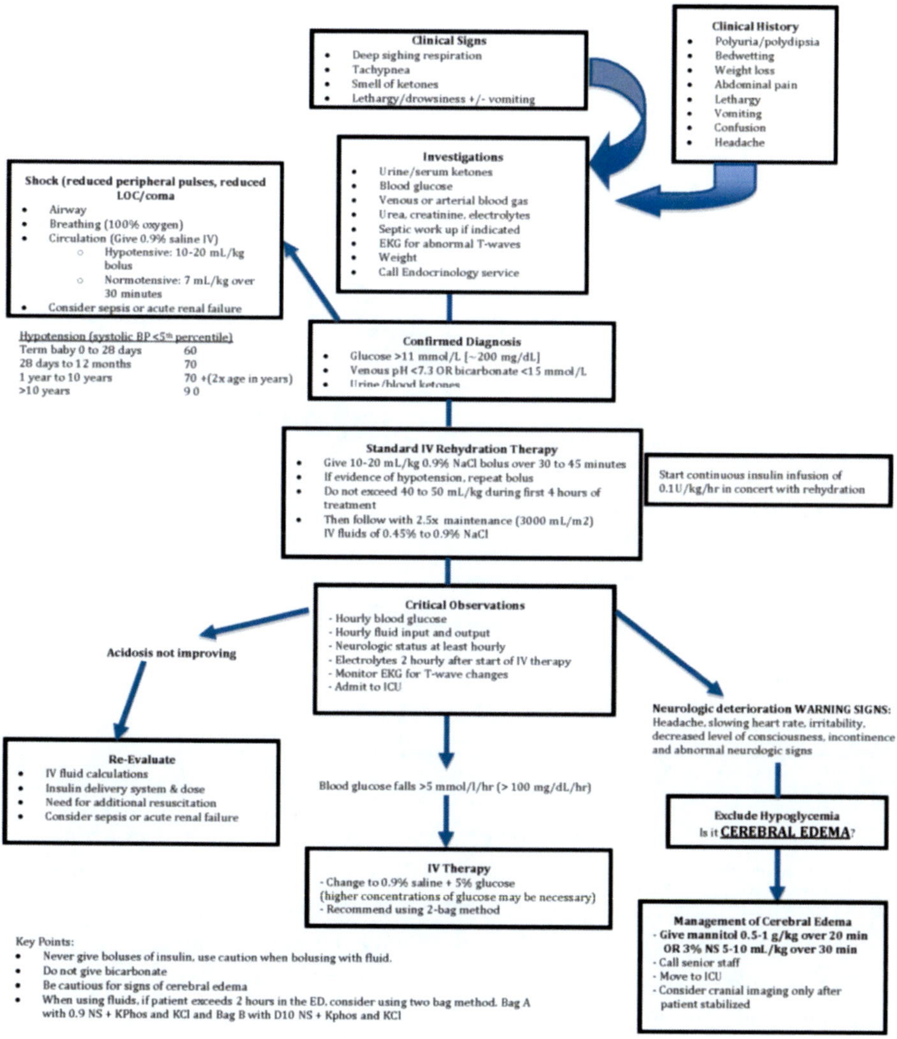

DIAGNOSIS AND ASSESSMENT

Patients with new onset diabetes presenting in DKA will typically present with the classic triad of polydipsia, polyuria, and weight loss over a prolonged period of time. Previously diagnosed patients tend to present more acutely. Patient complaints include abdominal pain, nausea, vomiting, and muscle pains or cramping. These signs and symptoms may be due to electrolyte imbalances and ketonemia. Later findings may include tachypnea or deep sighing breaths, (Kussmaul's respirations) compensating for metabolic acidosis and changes in mental status.

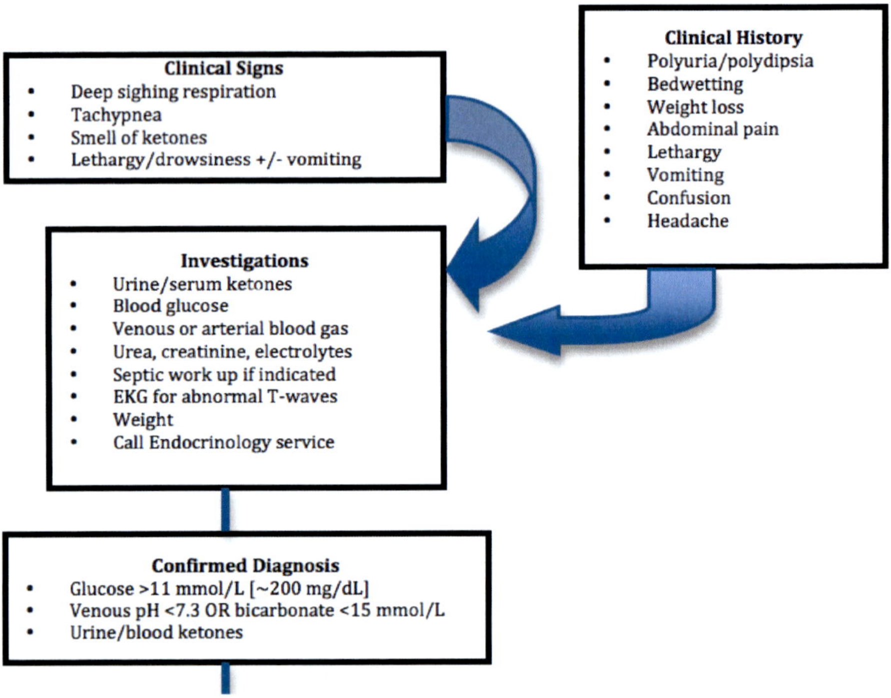

Diagnosis is confirmed by laboratory values: blood glucose concentration greater than 200 mg/dL, venous pH less than 7.3 or bicarbonate concentration less than 15 mmol/L and ketonuria and/or ketonemia.

Initial assessment of dehydration usually defines and directs appropriate orders for rehydration. Such assessment in nonacidotic children focuses on physical exam findings of capillary refill time, oral dryness, skin turgor and sunken fontanelle or eyes. However, none of these findings are reliable in predicting hydration in those patients with DKA. Olivieri and colleagues noted that acidosis can make a child seem more dehydrated due to tachypnea and mouth breathing, resulting in dry mucous membranes and vasoconstriction which may create cooler extremities. Evidence of tachycardia and orthostatic hypotension may also be present and are better predictors of true dehydration [1].

COMPONENTS OF MANAGEMENT

All patients with suspected DKA should have hourly monitoring of vital signs, neurologic status, blood glucose, and fluid balance [1].

There are three mainstays of DKA management: judicious rehydration, reversal of ketoacidosis and correction of electrolyte imbalance. Appropriate treatment of each of these pieces are important to avoid complication of DKA.

Rehydration is one of the most important factors in DKA management. It not only increases effective circulating blood volume and glomerular filtration rate (GFR), but also increases clearance of glucose and ketones. Initially, in patients who are normotensive, the preferred intravenous resuscitation is 10 to 20 mL/kg of Normal Saline (NS). This infusion may be repeated as needed for patients in hypovolemic shock. Thereafter, maintenance fluids should be initiated. Studies show there is no benefit of using colloid over crystalloid fluids and no data supports use of solutions more dilute than 0.45% NaCl [2]. In fact, many centers are advocating for the use of strictly isotonic fluids like NS in acutely ill patients. Thus, although adult management often includes hypotonic fluids, it is not considered pediatric best practice. This concept was not well recognized among many facilities in the Illinois ED study [3].

Standard IV Rehydration Therapy

- Give 10-20 mL/kg 0.9% NaCl bolus over 30 to 45 minutes
- If evidence of hypotension, repeat bolus
- Do not exceed 40 to 50 mL/kg during first 4 hours of treatment
- Then follow with 2.5x maintenance (3000 mL/m2) IV fluids of 0.45% to 0.9% NaCl

There are conflicting recommendations about the rate and volume of fluids needed, as defined by degree of patient dehydration. Felner and White studied fluid resuscitation in two groups of patients in the ED; the first with fluid deficit calculated by clinical determination of dehydration and the other using a standard volume regardless of clinical dehydration assessment. Overall, the second group received less fluid with no significant difference in time to resolution of metabolic acidosis [4]. This study documented that emergency departments can spend less time assessing extent of dehydration (physical exam findings and calculation of fluid deficit) and move more quickly to provide safe and expedited fluid resuscitation. The current best practice management for delivering dextrose is by use of the two-bag system. This method, as the name implies, involves two bags of fluid with identical electrolyte content but different dextrose contents that infuse simultaneously. The bags have 0% dextrose in one and 10% in the other to quickly titrate the amount of glucose given. For example, if using isotonic fluids, one bag would be D10NS and the other bag would be NS. Initially zero dextrose (NS) is administered as hyperglycemia in DKA resolves; this usually should occur while serum glucose is greater than 250 mg/dL. General guidelines advise giving roughly half of each bag to create 5% dextrose infusion when serum glucose is between 150 mg/dL and 250 mg/dL [1]. When the patient's glucose is less than 150 mg/dL, D10NS alone should be used while insulin continues to infuse. This system proved not only to save time, but has also been cost effective.

Because of the tendency of insulin to adsorb to plastic tubing, sufficient insulin should be infused throughout the entire IV tubing prior to the patient. While the rate of maintenance hydration is still under debate, the prevailing recommendations urge "correction" over 48 hours and at a rate "at or under $3L/m^2/day$.

The second important management factor is correction of ketoacidosis. This too involves fluid rehydration and insulin administration. Insulin is paramount in suppression of lipolysis and ketogenesis. "Low dose" continuous intravenous (IV) insulin is the standard of care using a rate of 0.1 units/kg/hour. A recent randomized controlled trial compared the use of insulin infusion rates of 0.1 units/kg/hour with 0.05 units/kg/hour and found no differences in time to resolution of acidosis or complications including hypokalemia, hypoglycemia or cerebral edema [5]. These investigators recommended further blinded superiority trials comparing the lower insulin infusion dose with the standard dose [5]. In contrast to adult patients, a bolus of insulin can be harmful to pediatric patients as it can increase the risks of hypoglycemia and cerebral edema [1]. According to data from ED practices in the State of Illinois, 33-43% of respondents would provide extra boluses of insulin following administration of insulin infusion; this practice is to be discouraged [3].

Start continuous insulin infusion of 0.1U/kg/hr in concert with rehydration

The insulin infusion should be continued until the pH is greater than 7.3, bicarbonate is greater than 20 mmol/L, and beta hydroxybutyrate is less than 1 mmol/L. The serum glucose goal is 200 mg/dL. Maintenance of glucose below renal threshold will minimize ongoing dehydration but must be monitored with extra care. When ketoacidosis resolves the patient is transitioned from the insulin infusion to subcutaneous insulin administration. This usually occurs after the patient has left the ED.

The third mainstay of DKA management is restoration of electrolyte imbalance of sodium, potassium and phosphate. A sodium deficit is the greatest of the three. Most practitioners use NS which allows for deficit replacement expeditiously. Noteworthy, is the fact that marked hyperglycemia induces an artificial depression in measured serum sodium (pseudohyponatremia). With appropriate insulin and fluid administration, the hyperglycemia improves; and this should be associated with a steady improvement in measured serum sodium. If such an improvement is not observed, at anytime in the treatment regimen, concern for fluid retention [similar to syndrome of inappropriate arginine vasopressin] must be raised and a decision to slow fluid administration rate is needed.

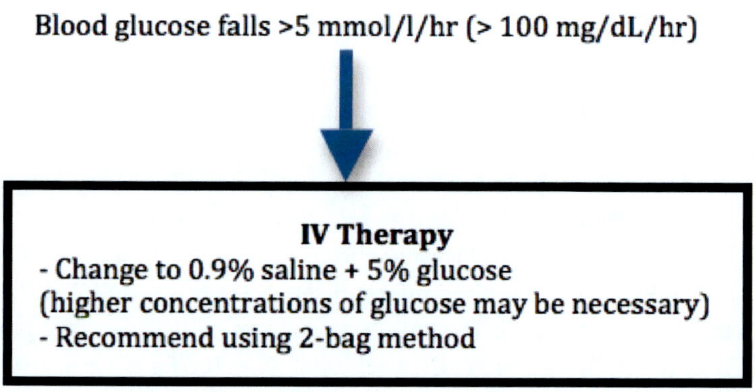

During the development of hyperglycemia and ketoacidosis, total body potassium will be decreased, though serum potassium measurements may be low, normal or high. The impact of insulin administration will direct potassium to reenter cells, resulting in decreased extracellular levels. It is important to monitor potassium not only before but also during insulin treatment. Use of continuous EKG monitoring allows for assessment of developing potassium toxicity: peaked T-waves for hyperkalemia and U-waves for hypokalemia.

Phosphate is also depleted due to osmotic diuresis in DKA. IV fluid administration and intracellular movement due to insulin administration can induce marked extracellular hypophosphatemia. Phosphate should be included in resuscitation fluids. Concentration of potassium phosphate supplementation should be kept no greater than 20 mEq/L in fluid rehydration solutions. Exceeding that concentration is associated with the development of clinical hypocalcemia.

All of these management components are best guided by a pediatric endocrinologist. Few facilities in Illinois had immediate access to a pediatric endocrinologist. In such an absence, the ED needs to have published state of the art consensus guidelines and protocols for DKA management. In Illinois, only 34% of EDs currently have protocols for DKA management.

POTENTIAL COMPLICATIONS

DKA management uniformly requires close monitoring. In a busy ED this can be a very difficult disease to manage. Many of the treatment factors are time sensitive and require a coordinated effort with cooperation between physicians and nursing staff. Such a reality makes movement out of the ED and into the appropriate in-patient management unit imperative.

However, the most devastating complication of DKA can still develop during the first few hours of treatment.

Cerebral edema may be present on admission from "home" or develop in the course of intervention. Onset to complete brain herniation may be rapid or slow. Deterioration in the Glasgow coma scale of 4 points is sufficient to presume the presence of cerebral edema until proven otherwise. Likewise, the sudden onset of headache or incontinence must raise the concern that cerebral edema is at hand. If not treated quickly, it can be fatal. If inappropriately treated, it may cause profound neurologic impairment. If anticipated and treated appropriately, the patient neurologic outcome is more likely to be favorable.

Clinically detectable cerebral edema is found in about one percent of episodes of DKA [7]. Glaser and colleagues found that preexisting risk factors included: elevation in BUN, marked depression in serum bicarbonate, co-treatment with sodium bicarbonate, and failure of measured serium sodium to elevate with therapy [6-10-9].

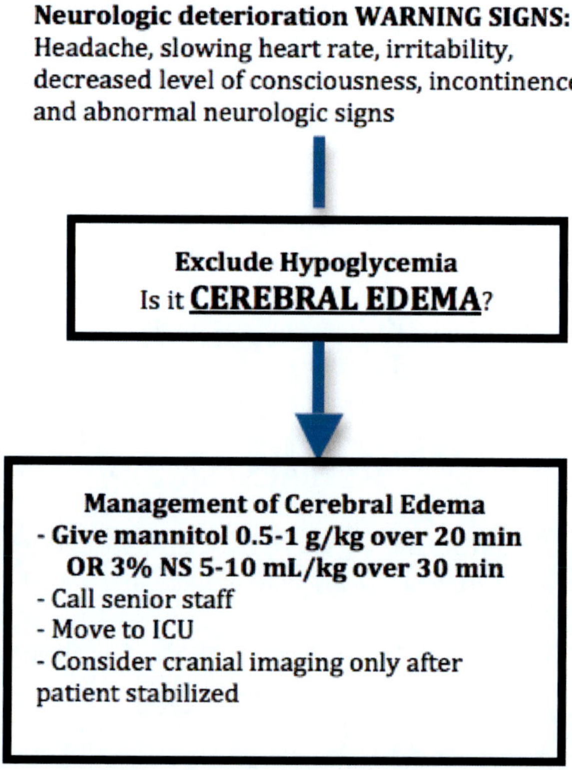

DISPOSITION FROM THE ED

Patients with mild DKA [bicarbonate > 20 mEq/L] will usually be able to be sent home directly from the emergency department. This mild state corrects after 2-3 hours of intravenous fluid hydration plus appropriate insulin administration. Follow up with the appropriate care provider is crucial. In established persons with diabetes mellitus, DKA is completely preventable!

Patients with moderate DKA (venous pH < 7.2; bicarbonate less than 10 mmol/L) or severe DKA (venous pH < 7.1; bicarbonate less than 5 mmol/L) need to be admitted to the hospital, and preferably a pediatric intensive care unit.

Conclusion

Evaluation and management of pediatric patients with DKA in the ED requires a well-organized effort by all caretakers. This is accomplished with expeditious but thoughtful fluid resuscitation, initiation of insulin infusion, and correction of metabolic acidosis and electrolyte imbalance. While many questions about best practice remain a matter of debate, we know a great deal about successful management of DKA in the pediatric ED. These well-documented protocols [see Flow chart] should represent best practice management in all emergency facilities to ensure the best care for patients with DKA.

References

[1] Olivieri, L. and Chasm, R. (2013). Diabetic ketoacidosis in the pediatric emergency department. *Emergency medicine clinics of North America*, 31(3), pp.755—773.

[2] Dunger, D., Sperling, M., Acerini, C., Bohn, D., Daneman, D., Danne, T., Glaser, N., Hanas, R., Hintz, R., Levitsky, L., Savage, M., Tasker, R. and Wolfsdorf, J. (2004). European Society for Paediatric Endocrinology/Lawson Wilkins Pediatric Endocrine Society Consensus Statement on Diabetic Ketoacidosis in Children and Adolescents. *PEDIATRICS*, [online] 113(2), pp.e133-e140. Available at: http://dx.doi.org/10.1542/peds.113.2.e133 [Accessed 2 Oct. 2014].

[3] Barrios, E., Hageman, J., Lyons, E., Janies, K., Leonard, D., Duck, S. and Fuchs, S. (2012). Current Variability of Clinical Practice Management of Pediatric Diabetic Ketoacidosis in Illinois Pediatric Emergency Departments. *Pediatric Emergency Care*, [online] 28(12), pp.1307-1313. Available at: http://dx.doi.org/10.1097/ pec.0b013e 3182768bfc [Accessed 2 Oct. 2014].

[4] Felner EI, White PC. Improving management of diabetic ketoacidosis in children. *Pediatrics* 2001;108:735-740.

[5] Nallasmy K, jayashree M, Singhi S Et al. Low dose vs standard dose insulin in pediatric diabetic ketoacidosis. *JAMA Pediatr* 2014;168:999-1005.

[6] Glaser, N., Barnett, P., McCaslin, I., Nelson, D., Trainor, J., Louie, J., Kaufman, F., Quayle, K., Roback, M., Malley, R. and others, (2001).

Risk factors for cerebral edema in children with diabetic ketoacidosis. *New England Journal of Medicine*, 344(4), pp.264--269.

[7] Bello, F., Sotos J.. Cerebral oedema in diabetic ketoacidosis in children. *Lancet* 1990;336:64.

[8] Duck, S., Wyatt, D. Factors associated with brain hernitation in the treatment of diabetic ketoacidosis. *Journal of Pediatrics* 1988;113:10-14.

[9] Harris, G., Fiordalisi, I., Finberg, L. Safe management of diabetic ketoacidemia. *Journal of Pediatrics* 1988;113:65-8.

[10] Harris, G., Fiordalisi, I., Harris, W., Mosovich, L., Finberg, L. Minimizing the risk of brain herniation during treatment of diabetic ketoacidemia: a retrospective and prospective study. *Journal of Pediatrics* 1990;117:22-31.

In: Pediatric Diabetic Ketoacidosis ISBN: 978-1-63483-220-5
Editors: S. C. Duck and J. R. Hageman © 2015 Nova Science Publishers, Inc.

Chapter 5

IN-HOSPITAL MANAGEMENT OF PEDIATRIC DIABETIC KETOACIDOSIS (DKA): PRESENTATION, DIAGNOSIS, AND TREATMENT*

Brandy Merritt[1], MD, Heather Fagan[2], MD, and Stephen C. Duck[3], MD

[1]Pediatrics and Pediatric Critical Care, University of South Alabama Children's and Women's Hospital, Mobile, AL, US
[2]Pediatric Critical Care, Nemours Children's Hospital, Orlando, FL, US
[3]Pediatric Endocrinology, NorthShore University HealthSystem, Evanston, IL, US

ABSTRACT

Failure to receive appropriate insulin therapy in a patient with type 1 diabetes mellitus (T1DM) results in diabetic ketoacidosis (DKA), a potentially fatal condition. DKA is defined as hyperglycemia, with a serum glucose concentration > 200 mg/dL, acidosis with pH < 7.3 and serum bicarbonate concentration < 15 mmol/L, and the presence of serum ketones.

Currently, no universal standard of care for treating pediatric patients presenting with DKA exists. Additionally, a wide range of subspecialists

* No financial disclosures for this paper.

and non-subspecialists are involved in treating pediatric patients with DKA resulting in a variety of treatment options. However, some generally accepted goals for treatment include the slow correction of hyperglycemia thereby slowly correcting serum osmolality, the slow correction of metabolic acidosis, as well as the correction of fluid and electrolyte derangements. Careful and precise management is imperative in an effort to avoid severe complications of DKA and its treatment including hypoglycemia, cerebral edema, permanent neurologic deficits and long-term memory or other neurologic dysfunction. In this chapter, aspects of management of pediatric patients with DKA after admission to the intensive care unit or pediatric acute care unit will be discussed.

Brief Review of Pathophysiology

Insulin is the hormone responsible for the intracellular transfer of glucose, and is secreted from the β cells of the pancreas [1]. The destruction of the β cells, most commonly from autoantibodies, results in insulin deficiency and T1DM [2]. The lack of insulin results in glucose that remains extracellular and thus is useless for energy production. Counter-regulatory hormones, such as glucagon, attempt to increase glucose production by glucogenolysis and gluconeogenesis [3]. Ongoing hyperglycemia leads to osmotic diuresis, electrolyte loss and dehydration [2]. Additionally, the body's cells are not able to take up the newly available glucose because of the continued lack of insulin, leading to further gluconeogenesis and hyperglycemia. This exacerbates the ongoing osmotic diuresis. As a result, cells ultimately rely on alternate pathways for energy production, such as lipolysis, or the breakdown of fatty acids. Lipolysis leads to ketogenesis [4]. Production of ketones, primarily acetoacetate and β-hydroxybutyrate, result in an overwhelmingly high anion gap metabolic acidosis [2].

Diabetic Ketoacidosis Definition and Severity:

- The diagnosis of DKA requires: hyperglycemia (> 200 mg/dL), elevated ketone body production, and metabolic acidosis (pH < 7.3 and/or serum bicarbonate level < 15 mmol/L) [5].
- The acidotic state must be documented by venous or arterial blood gas analysis plus assessment of serum beta-hydroxybutyrate concentration.

The severity of presentation may be "graded" based on the degree of acidosis:

- Mild DKA: venous pH from 7.2-7.3 or a serum bicarbonate < 15 mmol/L.
- Moderate DKA: venous pH 7.1-7.2 or a serum bicarbonate < 10 mmol/L.
- Severe DKA: venous pH < 7.1 or bicarbonate < 5 mmol/L [6].

As the severity increases, the need for pediatric intensive care management and monitoring, as well as the risk for significant morbidity and mortality of the disease and its treatment increase.

Disposition

Some individuals presenting in mild DKA will not require admission to the hospital. This is especially true if they are a patient with known T1DM rather than a child with a new diagnosis of the disease. In the former group, the expectation is that with 2-3 hours of appropriate fluid management and supplemental insulin administration the patient's nausea and vomiting will be controlled as well as their state of hydration and aberrant glucose excursion.

However, those presenting in moderate DKA would benefit from admission to an intensive care or acute care unit where high-acuity nursing and active physician oversight are provided.

A diagnosis of severe DKA necessitates admission to a facility capable of providing intensive care. Regardless of the location of the Intensive Care Unit (ICU), consultation with Pediatric Endocrinology is imperative.

Therapy and Consequences for Severe DKA: The Next 2 to 48 Hours

In practice, the patient transported to the ICU will already be diagnosed with DKA and have appropriate fluid and insulin therapy initiated. Additionally, initial laboratory analyses will likely be known and the patient's accurate intravenous intake and urinary output data analysis will be started.

In the emergency department [ED], as discussed in detail in a previous chapter, initial fluid therapy in patients not presenting with frank hypotension or hypovolemic shock should be isotonic Normal Saline or Lactated Ringer's solution at a volume of 10-20 ml/kg. Typically, regular or rapid acting biosynthetic insulin is started by the end of the first hour assuming that the change in glucose concentration has not been abnormally rapid causing a precipitous drop in serum osmolality. Continuous cardio-respiratory monitoring should be ongoing with hourly documentation of vital signs and neurological checks.

Maintenance Fluid: Type, Tonicity and Infusion Rates

As documented in the prior chapters, diabetic ketoacidosis in children is a condition marked by hyperosmolality and dehydration. Cautious and slow correction of both of these deficits is crucial, and requires frequent clinical examinations, laboratory evaluations and ongoing strict analysis of the patient intake and output.

Free water deficits are invariably greater than electrolyte losses, but both are noteworthy and will direct composition of maintenance fluid therapy.

The actual electrolyte losses vary due to duration and severity of disease. However, typical losses are as follows with the ranges noted in parentheses:

Water	30-100 ml/kg
Sodium	6 mmol/kg (5-13)
Potassium	5 mmol/kg (3-6)
Chloride	4 mmol/kg (3-9)
Phosphate	0.5-2.5 mmol/kg

The choice for maintenance fluid composition will reflect the physician's concerns for the slow correction of the patient's state of hyperosmolality. The correction is targeted to allow for lowering of serum osmolality at a rate no greater than 5 mOsm/hr. with a simultaneous reduction in serum glucose of < 100 mg/dl per hour [5.5mmol/L]. Thus, it is important to recognize that the patient in DKA has a relative pathologic hyperosmolality created by severe DKA. As a result, in the acute phase, it is recommended to administer isotonic fluids with potassium and phosphate so as not to give excessive "free water" via the administration of hypotonic fluid solutions.

Normal serum osmolality is generally measured as 278 – 300 mosm/L. Effective serum osmolality is increased by a factor of [Glucose (mg/dl) – 100]/ 18] in a patient with significant hyperglycemia. Best practice guidelines suggest correction of the fluid and electrolyte deficits over 36-48 hours. In practice, major academic centers recommend a broad range of "entire daily rates of fluid infusion":

~ 4000 ml/m^2	University of Texas Southwestern Medical Center, Dallas.
3175 ml/m^2	2006 American Diabetes Association Consensus Statement
2500 ml/m^2	Baylor College of Medicine, Houston, Texas. (personal communication)
1800 ml/m^2	University of Chicago Pritzker Medical School. (personal communication)

Normal fluid requirements are 1200-1500 ml/m^2/day, therefore some centers are quite cautious with regards to deficit replacement. In fact, few centers recommend replacing urine losses [output] during this phase of treatment. All centers advise choosing a replacement fluid rate that minimizes the risk of developing cerebral edema with isotonic fluid administration.

Several studies have been published demonstrating a "two bag system" to expedite bedside titration of intravenous dextrose concentrations [7]. This method involves one bag of intravenous fluids without dextrose (usually normal saline plus potassium and phosphate) and an identical bag of fluids with the addition of 10% dextrose (see Figure 1). A nurse-driven bedside protocol used for titration of a "two bag system" of IV fluids demonstrated an equivalent time to correction with equivalent safety profile. A "two bag system" can manipulate dextrose concentration with only two fluid bags, thereby avoiding a costly third bag of IV fluids (no dextrose, 5% dextrose and 10% dextrose) during acute correction [7].

At present, the International Society for Pediatric and Adolescent Diabetes (ISPAD) guidelines of 2014 acknowledge that no "rate of rehydration" can be considered superior to another. Having said that, rehydration rates of 1.5 – 2.0 times maintenance [2.25 – 3.0 L/m^2 daily] are commonly employed for the first 24 hours. Beyond the absolute rate of rehydration for many published protocols, individual centers will adjust the 24-48 hour time interval into smaller hourly intervals and alter fluid composition and osmolality in an effort to make slow and steady changes to glucose and osmolar concentrations as described above.

Further, the literature cautions not to exceed an infusion of 40 ml/kg during the first 4 hours of fluid therapy as this will undoubtedly drive a rapid osmolar shift increasing the pediatric patient's unique risk of cerebral compromise and cerebral edema.

Finally, the patient is to be kept on strict NPO during the duration of this acute treatment process.

INSULIN TREATMENT

Insulin therapy should be started by the end of the first hour of treatment for DKA. The standard of care currently is 0.1 unit/kg per hour. Bolus insulin therapy is definitively not recommended, and can be dangerous to the pediatric patient as the risk of an abrupt osmolar change is detrimental to the pediatric brain. This stands in stark contrast to the treatment of adult patients where the administration of bolus insulin is considered standard protocol in DKA management.

Further, careful attention to insuring "saturation" of the insulin infusion tubing by the drug is mandatory. Insulin is readily adsorbed onto the currently used IV tubing such that, failure to fully saturate the infusion tubing could delay actual delivery of insulin to the patient for hours at the slow infusion rate.

Recent publication suggests that lowering of insulin infusion rates to 0.05 unit/kg per hour will correct the metabolic derangements of DKA potentially as quickly and certainly as safely as the current standard [8, 9]. If a patient develops hypoglycemia during insulin therapy, this should be treated emergently with IV dextrose or oral juice or other oral glucose containing fluid if the patient is mentating appropriately to tolerate oral fluids without the risk of aspiration. Hypoglycemia that persists despite increases in the basal rate of dextrose may require decreasing the administration rate of insulin. However, as discussed in the chapter on the physiology of DKA, uncontrolled lipolysis is central to the biochemical imbalance. Consequently, suppression of lipolysis is paramount. The most sensitive of insulin actions is the suppression of lipolysis. Therefore, low but continuous insulin therapy is needed to emerge from the pathologic state of DKA. Thus, insulin therapy should only be discontinued in symptomatic hypoglycemia such as altered mental status or seizure.

Laboratory Monitoring

Glucose:

With the onset of dextrose free fluid rehydration, the measured glucose falls quickly. After the first 1-2 hours with the initial fluid "dilutional" decrease, serum glucose decreases should be no more rapid than 100 mg/dl [5.5 mmol/L] per hour.

The usual serum glucose value target during therapy is around 200-250mg/dl. This is a safe zone that should prevent hypoglycemia but is well above the renal threshold. In many centers, the implementation of the "2-bag" system of fluid and glucose delivery has effectively eliminated concern for hypoglycemia when the system is implemented correctly. With appropriate experience, the care team can maintain serum glucose in a more physiologic range, below renal threshold, and allow for more appropriate fluid balance during the resolution of ketoacidosis.

Monitoring of serum glucose should be obtained at the bedside every hour, and as part of a hospital laboratory panel at least every 4 hours. It is relatively common practice to institute dextrose containing fluids when the blood glucose falls below 200mg/dl to ensure that the child's glucose level remains safe, while being able to continue the insulin therapy.

Osmolality:

The need to reduce the patient's hyperosmolality slowly [< 5 mOsm/L hourly] is reported to reduce the risk of developing further cerebral swelling [see Chapter: Complications].

Sodium:

In conditions of marked hyperglycemia, serum sodium is artificially depressed. The degree is on the order of 1.6-2.4 mEq/L for every 100 mg/dl serum glucose above a baseline of 100 mg/dl. This is sometimes referred to as "pseudohyponatremia." The presence of excessive serum glucose exerts an osmotic effect and draws free water out of the cells into the serum. The result is a sodium level that appears artificially low on laboratory evaluation. With proper insulin and fluid administration, the serum sodium corrects in a steady, upward fashion. Failure to steadily improve the "corrected serum sodium" may be observed prior to the clinical development of cerebral edema. The normal control of arginine vasopressin is altered in pathologic states of DKA and can appear to create a state of inappropriate release [SIADH]. If that is the case, the concern for untoward fluid retention leading to cerebral edema should be appreciated, and fluid infusion rates should be abruptly decreased.

With the use of maintenance fluids that contain generous concentrations of sodium chloride, attention should be paid to the serum chloride concentration. With the resolution of ketoacidosis, the patient may be left with a hyperchloremic metabolic acidosis. However, this is typically of little physiologic significance, and thus should simply be recognized as the instigator for the mild metabolic acidosis that remains after correction of DKA.

Potassium:

Hyperkalemia as a condition is more likely to be evident upon presentation to the ED, but will resolve quickly with the initiation of insulin therapy which drives extracellular potassium to an intracellular position. In fact, the body is typically potassium depleted with the preexisting osmotic diuresis. However, to be safe, supplemental potassium should be withheld from the initial rehydration fluids until renal function is established with appropriate voiding.

By the time the patient reaches the in-patient unit, serum potassium will likely be in the low to normal range, and should be added to the maintenance infusion fluids as ongoing insulin administration will drive the extracellular potassium back into the intracellular spaces. Typically, potassium phosphate and/or potassium chloride are added to the intravenous fluids.

In the intensive care unit, the patient should be on continuous cardio respiratory and pulse oximetry monitoring

Phosphate and Calcium:

Serum phosphate will be driven into the intracellular spaces with insulin, leading to circulating hypophosphatemia. The patient will have total body phosphate depletion due to the preexisting osmotic diuresis in the disease state. Clinically, this electrolyte state is capable of decreasing the dissociation of oxygen off of hemoglobin, and could result in peripheral hypoxia. However, clinical trials have never established this as a credible concern. This is likely due to the prevailing ketoacidosis acting in the exact opposite fashion regarding the binding of oxygen to hemoglobin with increased oxygen delivery to the tissues.

As mentioned above, the use of chloride salts can create a metabolic acidosis following the resolution of ketoacidosis. Potassium phosphate is an excellent substitute for potassium chloride, for just such a reason. However, the concentration of phosphate supplementation should not exceed 20 mEq/L or a risk of tetany from hypocalcemia may occur with binding of the phosphate to the free calcium.

Beta-hydroxybutyrate and venous blood gas:

In the absence of cardiac compromise or cerebral edema, venous blood gas analysis, rather than arterial sampling, is sufficient. This data should be obtained every 2 hours for the first 12-24 hours, and then every 4 hours through resolution of the acute disease process. Following the initial rehydration in the ED, the measured pH and bicarbonate may be lower than on admission. Thereafter, steady increases in both are expected.

Clinical observation usually will document that the presence of Kussmaul respirations is associated with venous bicarbonate less than10 mEq/L, and that this pattern of breathing will resolve when the bicarbonate rises above 10 mEq/L.

Reagent strip assessment of beta-hydroxybutyrate [B-OHB] concentrations is available. These are more useful in the "at home" maintenance and monitoring of the person with diabetes. These bedside reagent strips are considered "normal" if < 0.6 mmol/L and elevated if > 1.5 mmol/L.

Hospital laboratory analysis of serum B-OHB confirms the existence of DKA if the value is > 7.0 mmol/L. As treatment proceeds, this concentration is expected to decrease steadily until it is absent or nearly absent with full resolution of the pathologic state.

Most children with DKA do not have compromised renal or cardiac function. Therefore the risk of lactic acidosis compounding ketoacidosis is not typical in the pediatric population. In DKA, the anion gap directly resulting from the ketoacidosis is typically 20-30 mmol/L. With a gap > 35 mmol/L, an element of lactic acidosis should definitively be considered.

Anion Gap =	$Na^+ - [Cl^- + HCO3^-]$

Renal function:

At presentation, the obligate dehydration will cause pre-renal azotemia with an increased serum urea nitrogen as compared to the elevation of creatinine. Assessment of renal function is necessary to exclude coexisting primary renal disease at presentation. Significant elevation in serum creatinine will alert the staff to carefully monitor serum potassium.

Accurate fluid Intake and Output:

It is mandatory that the patient be on strict oral fluid restriction, "nothing by mouth." The rapidity with which a thirsty child can drink fluids could severely impact the medical plan to correct fluid deficits slowly and meticulously over 36-48 hours.

With more conservative fluid resuscitation rates, an overall negative fluid balance may occur secondary to an osmotic diuresis from the glucose load during the initial stages of treatment. However, if a patient has evidence of hypovolemic shock, or hypotension, they should receive 10ml/kg of isotonic fluid imminently. Shock states place the patient at risk for decreased peripheral perfusion and untoward consequences of their aberrant hypercoagulation status in the face of critical illness. Further, sudden increased urine output, or the acute onset of diabetes insipidus should alert the physician to posterior pituitary compromise.

As treatment progresses, a positive fluid balance is expected, but if marked, the physician should consider decreasing the fluid infusion rate and more carefully assess neurologic status as this can be problematic as well.

Monitoring of Vital Signs

Age appropriate normal values for respiratory rate, heart rate and blood pressure

Age	Respiratory Rate (breaths per minute))	Heart Rate (beats per minute)	Blood Pressure (mm Hg)
Neonate	30-60	100-180	50-90
Infant [1 – 12 months]	24-50	100-160	60-100
Toddler [1 – 3 years]	24-40	90-150	80-105
Preschooler [3 – 5 years]	20-30	80-140	95-105
School age [5 – 12 years	10-30	65-120	95-120
Adolescent [> 12 years]	12-20	60-100	100-128

Monitoring of Neurological Signs

The pediatric DKA patient will present with variable levels of alertness related to their critical disease state, level of hydration, level of acidosis, and potential cerebral compromise. Hourly neurological and Glasgow Coma Scale (GCS) assessments are indicated in the ICU or acute care setting. Presentation with a GCS of < 14 or a decrease of 2 or more from the prior assessment should alert the physician to possible central nervous system compromise. As per the GCS criterion below, the best possible score is 15 while the worst is 3. The score is calculated by the combination of an eye, verbal and motor response. In the nonverbal child or toddler, there is an alternative way of assessing this "verbal" contribution to the overall score seen in the third column.

Glasgow Coma scale:

Best eye response	Best verbal response	Best in nonverbal toddler or child	Best motor response
Opens spontaneously = 4	Age appropriate interactions = 5	Smiles, orients, and follows = 5	Obeys commands = 6
On verbal command = 3	Disoriented and confused = 4	Consolable if crying, but interacts inappropriately = 4	Localizes pain, withdraws to touch = 5
On pain = 2	Verbal but incoherent = 3	Cries to pain, inconsistently consolable = 3	Withdraws to pain = 4
Not at all = 1	Only moans, sounds or groans = 2	Inconsolable, irritable, restless, moans = 2	Flexion to pain [decorticate posture] = 3
	No verbal response = 1	No response = 1	Extension to pain [decerebrate posture] = 2
			No response = 1

Onset of clinically significant cerebral edema [CE] and Neurologic Compromise:

As discussed in the chapter: Clinical Complications, the presence of cerebral brain swelling [edema] and increased intracranial pressure is common in pediatric patients with moderate to severe DKA upon presentation or in the acute states of treatment. In fact, the most serious and deadly complication associated with correction of DKA is cerebral edema. The incidence of clinical cerebral edema is approximated at 1% of total cases of DKA [10]. While the exact cause of the development of cerebral edema is unclear, several risk factors have been identified including: elevated blood urea nitrogen level (BUN), lower age at presentation, and the use of bicarbonate therapy [10].

Other risk factors for the development of cerebral edema also include: younger age, new onset, and a long duration of symptoms. Studies have shown that a substantial number of patients develop some degree of subclinical cerebral edema [10]. However, of those cases of clinically evident cerebral edema, 25% progress to death, 25% suffer severe neurologic disability, and the remainder recover. Cerebral edema may occur at any time during rehydration therapy, but most common develops several hours after the initiation of therapy [10]. If cerebral edema is suspected, it should be immediately treated with hypertonic saline or mannitol to imminently change the osmolar load. As noted above, the deterioration of Glasgow Coma scale scoring must be interpreted as impending cerebral crisis. The greatest majority of such crises are due to cerebral edema; the smaller minority is likely due to cerebral anoxia, ischemia or infarction.

The best bedside evaluation for acute CE is as follows [11]:

1. Any one of the 4 diagnostic criteria!
2. Any two major criteria: likely.
3. Any one major criterion and any two minor criteria: likely.

Diagnostic criterion	1. Decorticate or decerebrate posture 2. Cranial nerve palsy: especially 3,4, & 6 3. Abnormal neurogenic respiratory pattern. 4. Abnormal motor or verbal response to pain
Major criterion	1. Altered or fluctuating level of consciousness 2. Sustained cardiac deceleration > 20 bpm, not otherwise explained 3. Unexpected incontinence.
Minor criterion	1. Vomiting 2. Headache 3. Lethargy or stupor 4. Diastolic hypertension: > 90 mm Hg 5. Age < 5 years old

No patient should be removed from the intensive care unit for radiographic documentation of CE. Data does suggest that the CE is generalized and leads to bilateral, central transtentorial descending herniation with rostrocaudal brainstem compression. Whether suspected or "proven", acute CNS deterioration must be treated immediately. Consequently, the treatment agents are to be pre-ordered and at the bedside of any patient admitted in moderate to severe DKA. Awaiting delivery by pharmacy once the crisis developed is unacceptable. As a clinical caveat: if the patient was treated quickly and CE was not the cause, you likely merely delayed time to recovery; if the patient was treated quickly with CE with resolution of the symptoms, you likely saved not only his life but also the quality of his life. Another important clinical caveat is that even with careful and meticulous treatment and monitoring, some pediatric patients develop morbid CE that leads to significant compromise. Thus, as mentioned above, the entire pathophysiology of this devastating complication is still not clear.

The current principles of treatment include the following:

Current fluid infusion rate	Immediately reduce by a significant degree.
20% Mannitol [1100 mOsm/L]	0.25 to 1g/kg infused over 20 minutes; may be repeated after 30 minutes if no initial response
3% Sodium Chloride [1030 mOsm/L]	5 – 10 ml/kg over 10-15 minutes; may be repeated after 30 minutes if no initial response
Elevation of the head of the bed	The head should be elevated 30-45 degrees
Intubation and mechanical ventilation	Avoid hyperventilation with goal paCO2 35-40 mmHg. Hyperventilation will potentially cause arteriolar vasoconstriction and cerebral ischemia whereas hypoventilation may cause cerebral arteriolar vasodilation effectively increasing the intracranial pressure with increased arterial blood flow

Failure to recover quickly from the neurological complications of CE should lead to urgent consultation with Neurosurgery to further assess for the presence of increased intracranial pressure and neurologic dysfunction.

Transition out of the ICU to the General Ward

Pediatric patients with a pre-existing diagnosis of Type 1 diabetes mellitus develop severe DKA due to lack of appropriate treatment. While in the ICU, social work should be contacted to undertake a thorough family assessment to understand the reasons for this event. For the first several days post recovery, insulin resistance is likely significantly elevated such that "current or usual" pattern management profiles maybe insufficient. Patients newly diagnosed with Type 1 diabetes mellitus are usually sufficiently stable and recovered from the physiological aberrations of DKA so as to be moved to the general ward after 36 to 48 hours. Intense, new patient education will be required as part of the discharge process and will require additional inpatient or outpatient education depending on education resources at the institution. In the newly diagnosed patient, pre-existent hyperglycemia induces significant glucotoxicity and lipotoxicity. These require significantly more exogenous insulin to be administered during the initial 2-14 days of therapy. Control for the person with diabetes is best achieved by focusing on pattern management: the interplay of dietary intake, physical activity levels, and insulin administration.

Quality Improvement

Aspects of monitoring and management of DKA in the intensive care unit can be improved with a multidisciplinary "plan-do-study-act" quality improvement team approach. This has been accomplished by Merritt et al., in a project organized in a PICU setting [12] and by Koves and colleagues also in children's hospital setting [13]. Merritt's effort resulted in a decrease in patient costs when a comparison with pre-intervention costs was done [12]. The implementation of a DKA order-set utilizing the electronic medical record resulted in:

1. decreases in unanticipated hypokalemic episodes,
2. improvements in insulin infusion management was associated with reduced length of ICU stay,
3. overall improvement in DKA management and education,
4. cerebral edema occurrence and bicarbonate use were both reduced [13].

References

[1] Kumar et al. *Robbins and Cotran Pathologic Basis of Disease*. 7th edition (2005):1189-1205.

[2] Behrman et al. Nelson Textbook of Pediatrics. 17th edition (2004):1947-1972.

[3] Wolfsdorf J, Glaser N, Sperling M. Diabetic Ketoacidosis in Infants, Children, and Adolescents: A consensus statement from the American Diabetes Association. *Diabetic Care* 2006 May;29(5):1150-1159.

[4] Champe PC Harvey RA. *Biochemistry*. 2nd edition (1994):291-300.

[5] Kerr J, Moore M, Frank D, Gujral R. Management of Diabetic Ketoacidosis and Other Hyperglycemic Emergencies. *Society of Critical Care Medicine Critical Connections* 2012 6 Dec.

[6] Wolfsdorf JI et al. ISPAD Clinical Practice Consensus Guidelines 2014 Compendium: Diabetic Ketoacidosis and hyperglycemic hyperosmolar state. *Pediatric Diabetes* 2014;15(20):154-179.

[7] Poirier MP, Greer D, Satin-Smith. A prospective study of the "two-bag system" in diabetic ketoacidosis management. *Clin. Pediatr.* 2004;43(9):809-13

[8] Nallasamy K, Jayashree M, Singhi S, Bansai A. Low-Dose vs Standard-Dose Insulin in Pediatric Diabetic Ketoacidosis: A Randomized Clinical Trial. *JAMA Pediatr.* 2014 Nov 1;168(11):999-1005.

[9] Wolfsdorf JI. The International Society of Pediatric and Adolescent Diabetes guidelines for management of diabetic ketoacidosis: Do the guidelines need to be modified? *Pediatric Diabetes* 2014;15:277–286.

[10] Glaser N et al. Risk Factors for Cerebral Edema in Children with Diabetic Ketoacidosis. *N. Engl. J. Med.* 2001;344:264-269.

[11] Muir AB, Quisling RG, Yang MCK, et al Cerebral edema in childhood diabetic ketoacidosis, natural history, radiographic findings, and early identification, *Diabetes Care* 2004;27(7):1541 - 1546.

[12] Merritt BE et al. Protocol for the treatment of Pediatric Diabetic Ketoacidosis. *Poster Society of Critical Care Medicine*, Critical Care Congress 2013.

[13] Koves IH, et al. Improving care for pediatric diabetic ketoacidosis. *Pediatrics* 2014;134:e848-856.

In: Pediatric Diabetic Ketoacidosis ISBN: 978-1-63483-220-5
Editors: S. C. Duck and J. R. Hageman

Chapter 6

COMPLICATIONS AND OUTCOMES OF PEDIATRIC DIABETIC KETOACIDOSIS

G. Todd Alonso, MD
University of Colorado, Denver, CO, US
Barbara Davis Center for Childhood Diabetes, Aurora, CO, US

ABSTRACT

Diabetic ketoacidosis (DKA) is a frequent occurrence in diabetes mellitus. Despite advances in care, a small percentage of children suffer complications which can have devastating outcomes. The most common of these complications is cerebral edema. While contributing factors and mechanisms which predispose patients with DKA to cerebral edema are only partially understood, current consensus statements from professional societies such as the American Diabetes Association and the International Society for Pediatric and Adolescent Diabetes are able to provide clear guidance based on the best available evidence for optimizing outcomes in pediatric DKA.

INTRODUCTION

Diabetic ketoacidosis (DKA) is a complicated disease process characterized by many coexisting metabolic derangements. Absolute or relative insulin deficiency causes hyperglycemia, a resultant osmotic diuresis, and subsequent dehydration, hyperosmolarity, and electrolyte imbalances. Simultaneously, fatty acid breakdown leads to metabolic acidosis. Together, these factors put the patient at risk for organ damage which can cause permanent disability or death. Initiating appropriate therapy does not always guarantee an optimal outcome. Complications may arise during the hospital course, necessitating vigilance from the medical team. Many patients with DKA require the intensity and expertise available only in a critical care unit. For these reasons, the International Society for Pediatric and Adolescent Diabetes (ISPAD) recommends that children and adolescents who present with DKA be treated in centers with pediatric DKA experience where frequent monitoring of vital signs, neurological status, and laboratory assessments are possible. In cases where geography limits access to such a center, it is recommended that arrangements for telephone or videoconference support from a physician with experience with DKA be established.

A seven year retrospective study of pediatric DKA in the United Kingdom found that children with type 1 diabetes (T1D) have an overall mortality odds ratio (OR) of 2.3 compared to age matched controls [1]. An even higher mortality OR of 9.2 is noted among the 1 to 4 year old age group. Diabetic ketoacidosis was implicated in 82% of all deaths, and cerebral edema was present in at least 62% of all in-hospital deaths. Cerebral edema (CE-DKA) is the most common cause of death in patients with T1D.

Mortality for each episode of DKA ranges from 0.08 to 0.3%, with evidence of improving trends [1–4], likely a result of increased understanding of the inherent risks of DKA and the evolution of evidence based treatment protocols. Because CE-DKA is the major source of morbidity and mortality in pediatric DKA, many of the specific recommendations in DKA treatment algorithms are directed towards minimizing the occurrence and guiding the management of this frightening complication.

Cerebral Edema

Cerebral Edema – Epidemiology

Multicenter studies indicate that the incidence of clinically evident CE-DKA is 0.6-0.9% [5–7]. One retrospective series of 17 cases noted the timing of the identification of signs of brain swelling to range from as early as 180 minutes to as long as 30 hours after initiating therapy for DKA [8]. Others report evidence of CE-DKA even before intravenous therapy began. Cerebral edema is far less common in adults [9], although the protective factors that develop in older persons with T1D are not understood. Because CE-DKA is such a rare consideration in adult DKA, facilities with pediatric specific critical care will be the best equipped to care for these patients.

While CE-DKA is only diagnosed in a minority of pediatric patients, evidence of subclinical cerebral pathology has been detected in a majority of pediatric patients with DKA. Cranial computed tomography scans done prior to initiating therapy in seven of nine patients showed smaller lateral and third ventricles compared to the noted sizes in follow up scans seven days later. However, only one patient in that group was diagnosed with CE-DKA [10]. A study using cranial magnetic resonance imaging (MRI) also found ventricular narrowing in 22 of 42 pediatric patients with DKA [11]. Cerebral oximetry evaluation in 19 patients with DKA aged 8 to 18 years revealed that 90% had evidence of cerebral hyperemia as early as the second hour of treatment which persisted beyond 24 hours in at least four [12]. Therefore, subclinical CE-DKA is a common phenomenon, albeit of uncertain significance.

Cerebral Edema – Pretreatment Factors

Multiple pretreatment factors are associated with increased odds of developing CE-DKA. Most indicate that patients with more severe metabolic derangements have higher risk. Lower initial HCO_3 [7] and PCO_2 [5, 11, 13], as well as higher initial serum urea [5, 7, 11, 13, 14] and glucose concentrations [7, 13] suggest that greater degrees of acidosis and dehydration at presentation predispose patients with DKA to develop brain swelling. Retrospective analysis of 34 CE-DKA cases demonstrated that the risk for development of CE-DKA was threefold higher in patients with new onset diabetes compared to those with established diabetes (11.9 vs 3.8 per 1000) [6]. The reasons for this difference are not clear. Younger age is also associated with a greater risk of cerebral edema [5, 15]. Therefore, most experts agree that younger age, new onset diabetes, and more severe initial laboratory assessment increase risk for CE-DKA, and admission to pediatric critical care should be considered [16].

Neuroinflammation appears to be an important event in the development of CE-DKA. Pathologic examination of cerebral tissue from fatal cases of CE-DKA revealed increased expression of proinflammatory mediators and disruption of vascular tight junctions, leading to structural and functional alteration of blood brain barrier integrity [17]. The albumin extravasation observed in these cases would decrease the relative serum oncotic pressure, and thus potentiate vasogenic edema in the brain. A vasogenic rather than a cytotoxic process is further supported by elevated apparent diffusion coefficients on cerebral MRI [11] and by multiple reports of rapid neurological improvement with the intravenous infusion of mannitol or hypertonic saline [18]. Despite all the known associations in CE-DKA, no unified theory sufficiently explains the complicated etiology that predisposes these patients to brain swelling.

Cerebral Edema – Treatment Factors

Knowing that patients with DKA are dehydrated, thirsty, and tachycardic, the temptation is to aggressively administer intravenous (IV) fluid as though treating hypovolemic shock. However, earlier studies indicated that dramatically greater rates of IV rehydration were associated with increased risk of developing CE-DKA [19]. Patients presenting with DKA have increased osmolarity throughout the body from elevated sodium, glucose, and urea concentrations which developed over hours to days. Therefore, a treatment induced rapid drop in serum osmolarity due to the administration of relatively hypotonic IV fluids was hypothesized to be a major driving force behind CE-DKA. Whereas quickly decreasing serum osmolarity would occur in minutes, the blood brain barrier prevents an equally rapid adjustment, leading to free water influx into the brain tissue.

Although two pediatric DKA studies failed to show an association between CE-DKA and total fluid volume administered [5, 20], larger IV fluid volume in the first four to eight hours of DKA management was associated with an increased CE-DKA risk [20, 21]. Additionally, in a review of 12 CE-DKA cases, patients were more likely to have experienced not only a larger decrease in effective plasma osmolarity early in the course of therapy, but also to have had higher urine output and a more positive fluid balance [21]. Therefore, while the question of optimal IV fluid rate and content is still outstanding, most pediatric DKA protocols restrict initial IV fluid boluses to 10-20 mL/kg, reserve further boluses for signs of shock, and propose limits to ongoing IV hydration to minimize the risk of CE-DKA [16]. When treating a patient with DKA, it is important for the clinician to recall that in addition to dehydration, the acidosis is also a strong stimulator of tachycardia. Only a minimal decrease in heart rate is noted in the first hour of rehydration, regardless the volume of fluid given.

Notwithstanding cautious fluid management, other data suggest the genesis of CE-DKA is very complicated. As discussed above, brain swelling prior to the administration of IV fluids is common. A retrospective analysis of the causes of death in pediatric patients with T1D found that eight of the 24 out-of-hospital deaths in those with probable or definite DKA had brain swelling on postmortem examination. Taken together, 5-19% of pediatric patients with DKA have clinical findings of brain swelling prior to receiving IV fluid therapy [5, 7, 22–24]. Therefore, IV fluid content and rate cannot fully explain the development of CE-DKA.

In 2013 White and Dickson reported a rate of CE-DKA of only 0.5% in 3712 DKA admissions at a single center. No deaths from CE-DKA occurred [3]. Their protocol used IV hydration rates about 30% greater than those outlined in recent consensus statements [16, 25, 26]. The authors suggested that their favorable outcomes may be partly attributable to use of 0.675% NaCl, which provided a higher tonicity to the maintenance fluid and may satisfy an ideal tonicity for DKA resuscitation. Ongoing studies are expected to identify an optimal fluid and electrolyte replacement protocol in DKA.

Insulin administration in the first hour of therapy has been associated with increased odds of developing CE-DKA [20]. Further study found it to be more likely in patients who received an IV insulin bolus early in therapy than in those who did not [21]. Because of these data and the fact that blood glucose drops quickly with the initial IV fluid bolus, experts agree that an IV insulin bolus is unnecessary and perhaps even dangerous in DKA.

Limited data exists regarding an association between bicarbonate administration in DKA and the risk of CE-DKA. A 2011 systematic review found three pediatric nonrandomized studies addressing the question [27] (p20). In a multicenter case-control study involving 61 children with CE-DKA administration of bicarbonate was the only treatment factor associated with a greater risk (relative risk 4.2) of cerebral swelling when compared with matched controls [5]. Two smaller studies found a trend towards a similar association, but the effect was nonsignificant after controlling for covariates [7, 20].

Additionally, bicarbonate use in DKA has been associated with a paradoxical increase in cerebrospinal acidosis that could exacerbate hypokalemia. Among the most severely acidotic patients (initial pH < 6.85), controlled trials have failed to show any clinical benefit from bicarbonate therapy. Published data are quite limited. For all of these reasons, while ISPAD does not proscribe the administration of IV bicarbonate, their consensus statement does include a cautious warning about its use [16].

Whereas one of the traditional therapies for cerebral edema was airway intubation with hyperventilation, current evidence indicates that it could actually be counterproductive in the treatment of DKA. Hyperventilation has the potential to decrease brain swelling via arterial autoregulation. Decreasing pCO_2 leads to cerebral artery constriction and therefore less hydrostatic pressure, allowing free water to travel out of the brain parenchyma. However, in a review of 61 cases of CE-DKA from 10 centers, hyperventilation was associated with poorer neurologic prognosis [14]. The authors speculate that decreased cerebral blood flow contributes to cerebral ischemia, potentially exacerbating evolving brain injury. Thus, intubation and mechanical ventilation should be reserved for impending respiratory failure. A review involving 85% of tertiary care pediatric hospitals in the US found that 17.8% of CE-DKA patients were mechanically ventilated [4]. Respiratory arrest in the setting of CE-DKA carries a very poor prognosis [6].

Cerebral Edema – Diagnosis

Patients may develop symptoms of CE-DKA any time from before presentation to the hospital to as late as 30 hours following initiation of therapy [8]. Clinical findings range from nonspecific changes in mental status such as somnolence or irritability to obvious signs of cerebral herniation (Table 1). A review of 26 cases of severe CE-DKA and 69 episodes of uncomplicated DKA was used to develop a bedside evaluation protocol with a 92% sensitivity and 4% false positive rate [8]. At least one diagnostic criterion was positive in all cases, and included abnormal response to pain, decorticate or decerebrate posturing, cranial nerve palsy (especially III, IV, and VI), and abnormal respiratory pattern (e.g., grunting, tachypnea, Cheyne-Stokes respiration, apneusis). Cranial nerve palsies and papilledema are specific neurological signs caused directly by increased intracranial pressure. As pressure inside the cranial vault increases, the sympathetic nervous system is stimulated, resulting in constriction of the body's arterioles and thereby causing hypertension. Increased blood pressure then stimulates baroreceptors in the aortic arch, triggering a parasympathetic response which slows the heart rate. Usually late signs, the development of hypertension and bradycardia during treatment for DKA are grave indicators.

Table 1. Clinical findings in 34 cases of CE-DKA [6]

Reduced level of consciousness	100%
Hypertension and bradycardia	41%
Pupil abnormalities	35%
Decerebrate or decorticate posturing	15%
Respiratory arrest	29%

Early recognition and treatment of CE-DKA is critical. A review of 69 cases found that over half of the 23 in whom therapy for the brain swelling was initiated early survived intact or disabled. Only 3 of the 46 who were treated late or not at all survived [15].

Neuroimaging has an unsatisfactory sensitivity for identification of CE-DKA. Glaser et al., showed that a brain CT could be normal even after the development of the first signs of CE-DKA [8, 28]. Moreover, a CT scan requires the patient to be out of the intensive care unit. Therefore, the physician should rely primarily on clinical diagnosis. Therapy for clinically suspected CE-DKA should not be delayed for cranial imaging. As discussed below, emergent brain CT may be considered in a critically ill patient with encephalopathy or acute focal neurologic deficit for the identification of a lesion which requires emergency neurosurgery (e.g., intracranial hemorrhage) or anticoagulation (e.g., cerebrovascular thrombosis) [16].

Cerebral Edema – Treatment

Because of the known association between IV fluids and CE-DKA, fluid rate should be decreased and the head of the bed elevated 30 degrees as soon as CE-DKA is suspected. Hyperosmolar IV fluids should be available at the bedside and administered without delay. In the past, mannitol, a nonmetabolized sugar alcohol, was the usual agent considered for the treatment of CE-DKA. However, 3% hypertonic saline more recently became an acceptable alternative [29], possibly because of easier storage at the bedside. Though the mechanism is unclear, both agents are believed to improve cerebral blood flow through decreased blood viscosity and reducing the intracellular volume via osmotic effects on the brain neurons [4]. Many observers cite rapid improvement in patients' clinical status upon administration of either agent.

In a review of over 43,000 pediatric DKA cases throughout the United States from 1999 to through 2009, 3.8% of patients were treated with hyperosmolar therapy. Most received mannitol as a sole agent, but 3% sodium chloride infusion increased during that time [4]. The authors called for clinical equipoise regarding the use of one agent over the other because of higher mortality (adjusted odds ratio 2.71) when 3% saline was used alone. This will need to be investigated with a prospective trial.

Cerebral Edema – Outcome

CE-DKA was the identified cause for 50 to 60% of diabetes related deaths in children [1, 15]. The mortality for patients with CE-DKA is now reduced to 21-24% [5–7, 14]. In addition, 57 to 65% of CE-DKA survivors have no long-term neurologic sequelae [5, 6, 14]. Persistent neurologic deficits in CE-DKA survivors include motor deficits, visual impairment, short term memory loss, dysphasia, dysarthria, and learning and emotional problems.

Other Conditions Complicating DKA

After CE, a variety of other problems account for the remaining morbidity and mortality in pediatric DKA. Each of these conditions is relatively rare and much less thoroughly studied in DKA than CE, though enough literature exists to aid clinicians' decision-making.

Hypercoagulability/Thrombosis

Reports of cerebral and deep venous thromboses indicate that DKA is a hypercoagulable state. Dehydration, osmolarity, tissue hypoxia, acidosis, and hyperlipidemia are some of the factors which have been proposed to promote thrombosis in these patients. Coagulation assessment in DKA demonstrated transiently increased von Willebrand Factor and decreased levels of protein C and decreased activity of protein S [30] in patients with no underlying clotting abnormalities. Some patients who experience severe thrombotic events during DKA have been found to have underlying hypercoagulable disorders such as sickle trait [3] and protein S deficiency [31]. Acute, focal neurologic deficits, seizures, decerebrate posturing, hemiparesis, or respiratory failure during an episode of DKA should raise suspicion for cerebral thrombosis, and brain imaging may be appropriate.

A case control study in children who underwent femoral venous catheterization during DKA indicated an increased risk for deep venous thrombosis when compared to other children in shock [32]. The risk was especially high for infants and toddlers. The authors suggest that a thrombosis prophylaxis regimen would be rational in this population.

Potassium Derangements

Abnormal serum potassium levels are very common in DKA. Dehydration leads to avid renal sodium retention through the renin/angiotensin/aldosterone pathway at the expense of a large urinary potassium loss. However, as most of the body's potassium is intracellular, serum potassium measurements do not reflect the state of depletion, and therefore patients may present with hyper-, normo-, or hypo-kalemia. Insulin administration shifts potassium intracellularly, potentially causing a dangerous degree of hypokalemia. In their series, Glaser et al., reported two deaths from hypokalemia and hypocalcemia which led to cardiac arrest [5]. The authors advise that patients have continuous electrocardiographic (ECG) monitoring of lead II if the initial serum potassium level is ≤3 mEq/L or ≥6 mEq/L. ECG abnormalities seen in the setting of abnormal potassium levels are shown below:

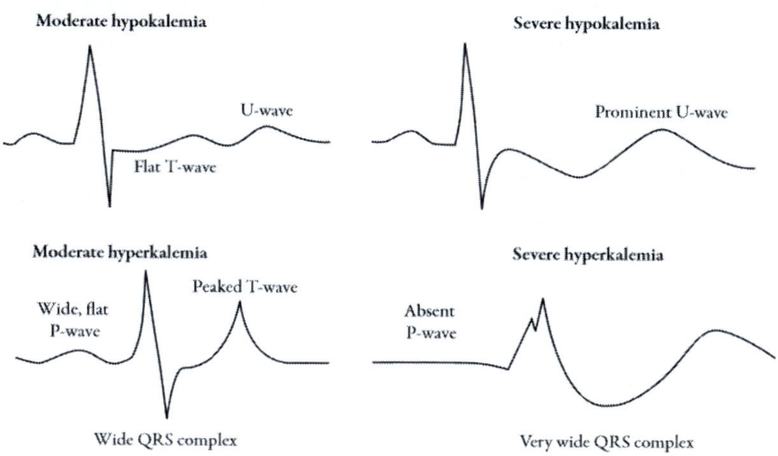

Figure 1. Electrocardiographic patterns for hypo- and hyperkalemia [33].

If hypokalemia causes severe ECG changes, insulin therapy should be withheld until sufficient potassium can be administered, and then insulin can be infused at a slower rate [34].

Hypophosphatemia

The osmotic diuresis of evolving DKA also causes phosphate loss. Insulin therapy drives phosphate intracellularly, potentiating hypophosphatemia. Severe hypophosphatemia is rare, but can lead to metabolic encephalopathy, seizure, impaired myocardial contractility, respiratory failure, dysphagia, ileus, hemolysis, and rhabdomyolysis, and reduced oxygen release from hemoglobin [16]. Overly aggressive IV phosphate replacement can lead to hypocalcemia. Small, prospective studies failed to show benefit of phosphate replacement during DKA therapy [16], but most centers administer some phosphate in their DKA resuscitation fluids.

Cardiac Arrhythmias

A prolonged QTc interval occurs frequently during DKA and correlates with the level of ketosis [35]. Additionally, T wave inversion has also been reported during DKA in the setting of normokalemia, which the authors postulate could be due to tachycardia or hyperventilation leading to poor coronary artery filling [36].

Rhabdomyolysis

Rhabdomyolysis is a relatively common complication in patients presenting with hyperglycemic hyperosmolar state, but far more infrequent in DKA [33]. Myoglobinuria will not necessarily cause darkened urine, and laboratory tests for myoglobinuria lack sensitivity [37]. Therefore, muscular weakness accompanied by low phosphate or potassium levels should raise suspicion for rhabdomyolysis. Renal failure, also very rare in pediatric DKA, is associated with rhabdomyolysis and should prompt consideration of dialysis [33].

Pancreatitis

Acute pancreatitis is diagnosed in about 2% of children with DKA, whereas the incidence is closer to 10% in adults [38]. Elevations in serum amylase and lipase are much more common, present in 40% of pediatric DKA [38]. Most of the amylase is believed to be from salivary origin, and the lipase level is directly associated with the degree of acidosis [33]. Therefore, providers should evaluate a patient for pancreatitis when abdominal pain is greater than expected for the clinical condition or does not abate with standard DKA therapy.

About 40% of children with DKA have elevated triglycerides, but the levels are usually not in the range expected to lead to acute pancreatitis (> 1000 mg/dL) [38]. Plasmapheresis has been used successfully to treat severe hypertriglyceridemia in a child with DKA and pancreatitis [39]. Patients who present with severe triglyceride elevations do not necessarily have familial hypertriglyceridemia [40].

Infections

Patients with DKA may be at increased risk of infection, but sepsis appears to be exceedingly rare in this group. During DKA, neutrophils have impaired chemotaxis and are less able to generate reactive oxygen species [41]. Mucormycosis is a rare, opportunistic infection experienced by a very small number of patients with DKA, but it is associated with a grave prognosis [33]. One series indicated a mortality rate of 40% when there was cerebral involvement [42].

Pulmonary Edema

Acute pulmonary edema and adult respiratory distress syndrome have been reported in children with DKA [43]. Pulmonary CT scans in children with DKA demonstrated interstitial pulmonary edema, even very early in therapy [10]. The mechanisms for these findings are unclear, but could represent pathology similar to cerebral edema.

Neurocognitive Effects

Although overall intellectual abilities in children with T1D are typically normal, there are detectable deficits in memory performance [44, 45]. In the past, most of the concern for neurocognitive deficits in patients with T1D focused on the effects of hypoglycemia [46], but there is now growing evidence that DKA events are associated with disrupted memory function [47, 48].

Conclusion

Diabetic ketoacidosis represents a dangerous set of metabolic abnormalities brought about by insulin deficiency leading to hyperglycemia, osmotic diuresis, and acidosis. While there are many potential complications in DKA therapy, cerebral edema is by far the most dangerous. Fortunately, modern DKA therapy results in complete recovery for almost all patients. Key principles for optimal outcomes include judicious fluid and electrolyte replacement, close monitoring of clinical signs and laboratory assessments, and treatment in a facility with the expertise and tools to provide appropriate therapy and manage complications.

References

[1] Edge JA, Ford-Adams ME, Dunger DB. Causes of death in children with insulin dependent diabetes 1990–96. *Arch. Dis. Child.* 1999;81(4):318-323.

[2] Curtis JR, To T, Muirhead S, Cummings E, Daneman D. Recent Trends in Hospitalization for Diabetic Ketoacidosis in Ontario Children. *Diabetes Care*. 2002;25(9):1591-1596. doi:10.2337/diacare.25.9.1591.

[3] White PC, Dickson BA. Low Morbidity and Mortality in Children with Diabetic Ketoacidosis Treated with Isotonic Fluids. *J. Pediatr.* 2013;163(3):761-766. doi:10.1016/j.jpeds.2013.02.005.

[4] DeCourcey DD, Steil GM, Wypij D, Agus MSD. Increasing Use of Hypertonic Saline Over Mannitol in the Treatment of Symptomatic Cerebral Edema in Pediatric Diabetic Ketoacidosis: An 11-Year Retrospective Analysis of Mortality*. *Pediatr Crit. Care Med.* 2013;14(7):694-700. doi:10.1097/PCC.0b013e3182975cab.

[5] Glaser N, Barnett P, McCaslin I, et al. Risk factors for cerebral edema in children with diabetic ketoacidosis. *N. Engl. J. Med.* 2001;344(4):264-269.

[6] Edge JA, Hawkins MM, Winter DL, Dunger DB. The risk and outcome of cerebral oedema developing during diabetic ketoacidosis. *Arch. Dis. Child.* 2001;85(1):16-22.

[7] Lawrence SE, Cummings EA, Gaboury I, Daneman D. Population-based study of incidence and risk factors for cerebral edema in pediatric diabetic ketoacidosis. *J. Pediatr.* 2005;146(5):688-692. doi:10.1016/j.jpeds.2004.12.041.

[8] Muir AB, Quisling RG, Yang MCK, Rosenbloom AL. Cerebral Edema in Childhood Diabetic Ketoacidosis Natural history, radiographic findings, and early identification. *Diabetes Care.* 2004;27(7):1541-1546. doi:10.2337/diacare.27.7.1541.

[9] Azzopardi J, Gatt A, Zammit A, Alberti G. Lack of evidence of cerebral oedema in adults treated for diabetic ketoacidosis with fluids of different tonicity. *Diabetes Res. Clin. Pract.* 2002;57(2):87-92.

[10] Hoffman WH, Steinhart CM, Gammal T el, Steele S, Cuadrado AR, Morse PK. Cranial CT in children and adolescents with diabetic ketoacidosis. *Am. J. Neuroradiol.* 1988;9(4):733-739.

[11] Glaser NS, Wootton-Gorges SL, Buonocore MH, et al. Frequency of sub-clinical cerebral edema in children with diabetic ketoacidosis. *Pediatr Diabetes.* 2006;7(2):75-80. doi:10.1111/j.1399-543X. 2006.00156.x.

[12] Glaser NS, Tancredi DJ, Marcin JP, et al. Cerebral Hyperemia Measured with Near Infrared Spectroscopy during Treatment of Diabetic Ketoacidosis in Children. *J. Pediatr.* 2013;163(4):1111-1116. doi:10.1016/j.jpeds.2013.06.008.

[13] Fiordalisi I, Novotny WE, Holbert D, Finberg L, Harris GD. An 18-yr prospective study of pediatric diabetic ketoacidosis: an approach to minimizing the risk of brain herniation during treatment. *Pediatr Diabetes.* 2007;8(3):142-149. doi:10.1111/j.1399-5448.2007.00253.x.

[14] Marcin JP, Glaser N, Barnett P, et al. Factors associated with adverse outcomes in children with diabetic ketoacidosis-related cerebral edema. *J. Pediatr.* 2002;141(6):793-797. doi:10.1067/mpd.2002.128888.

[15] Rosenbloom AL. Intracerebral crises during treatment of diabetic ketoacidosis. *Diabetes Care.* 1990;13(1):22-33. doi:10.2337/ diacare. 13.1.22.

[16] Wolfsdorf JI, Allgrove J, Craig ME, et al. Diabetic ketoacidosis and hyperglycemic hyperosmolar state. *Pediatr Diabetes*. 2014;15(S20):154-179. doi:10.1111/pedi.12165.
[17] Hoffman WH, Stamatovic SM, Andjelkovic AV. Inflammatory mediators and blood brain barrier disruption in fatal brain edema of diabetic ketoacidosis. *Brain Res*. 2009;1254:138-148. doi:10.1016/j.brainres.2008.11.100.
[18] Tasker RC, Acerini CL. Cerebral edema in children with diabetic ketoacidosis: vasogenic rather than cellular? *Pediatr Diabetes*. 2014;15(4):261-270. doi:10.1111/pedi.12153.
[19] Duck S, Wyatt D. Factors associated with brain herniation in the treatment of diabetic ketoacidosis. *J. Pediatr*. 1988;113(1):10-14.
[20] Edge JA, Jakes RW, Roy Y, et al. The UK case–control study of cerebral oedema complicating diabetic ketoacidosis in children. *Diabetologia*. 2006;49(9):2002-2009. doi:10.1007/s00125-006-0363-8.
[21] Hoorn EJ, Carlotti APCP, Costa LAA, et al. Preventing a Drop in Effective Plasma Osmolality to Minimize the Likelihood of Cerebral Edema During Treatment of Children with Diabetic Ketoacidosis. *J. Pediatr*. 2007;150(5):467-473. doi:10.1016/j.jpeds.2006.11.062.
[22] Couch RM, Acott PD, Wong GW. Early Onset Fatal Cerebral Edema In Diabetic Ketoacidosis. *Diabetes Care*. 1991;14(1):78-79. doi:10.2337/diacare.14.1.78b.
[23] Glasgow AM. Devastating Cerebral Edema in Diabetic Ketoacidosis Before Therapy. *Diabetes Care*. 1991;14(1):77-78. doi:10.2337/diacare.14.1.77.
[24] Warncke K, Dressel P, Ziegler A-G, et al. Severe Pretreatment Cerebral Edema in Newly Diagnosed Type 1 Diabetes. *Horm. Res. Paediatr*. 2014. doi:10.1159/000357140.
[25] Dunger DB, Sperling MA, Acerini CL, et al. European Society for Paediatric Endocrinology/Lawson Wilkins Pediatric Endocrine Society Consensus Statement on Diabetic Ketoacidosis in Children and Adolescents. *Pediatrics*. 2004;113(2):e133-e140. doi:10.1542/peds.113.2.e133.
[26] Wolfsdorf J, Craig ME, Daneman D, et al. Diabetic ketoacidosis in children and adolescents with diabetes. *Pediatr Diabetes*. 2009;10:118-133. doi:10.1111/j.1399-5448.2009.00569.x.
[27] Chua HR, Schneider A, Bellomo R. Bicarbonate in diabetic ketoacidosis - a systematic review. *Ann. Intensive Care*. 2011;1:23. doi:10.1186/2110-5820-1-23.

[28] Glaser NS, Wootton-Gorges SL, Buonocore MH, et al. Subclinical Cerebral Edema in Children With Diabetic Ketoacidosis Randomized to 2 Different Rehydration Protocols. *Pediatrics*. 2013;131(1):e73-e80. doi:10.1542/peds.2012-1049.

[29] Curtis JR, Bohn D, Daneman D. Use of hypertonic saline in the treatment of cerebral edema in diabetic ketoacidosis (DKA). *Pediatr Diabetes*. 2001;2(4):191.

[30] Carl G, Hoffman W, Passmore G, et al. Diabetic Ketoacidosis Promotes a Prothrombotic State. *Endocr. Res*. 2003;29(1):73.

[31] Sdogou T, Kossiva L, Kakleas K, et al. Deep Vein Thrombosis and Pulmonary Embolism in a Child with Diabetic Ketoacidosis and Protein S Deficiency: A Case Report. *Horm Res. Paediatr*. 2013;79(2):114-118. doi:10.1159/000343813.

[32] Gutierrez JA, Bagatell R, Samson MP, Theodorou AA, Berg RA. Femoral central venous catheter-associated deep venous thrombosis in children with diabetic ketoacidosis. *Crit. Care Med*. 2003;31(1):80-83.

[33] Rosenbloom AL. The management of diabetic ketoacidosis in children. *Diabetes Ther*. 2010;1(2):103-120. doi:10.1007/s13300-010-0008-2.

[34] Davis SM, Maddux AB, Alonso GT, Okada CR, Mourani PM, Maahs DM. Profound hypokalemia associated with severe diabetic ketoacidosis. *Pediatr Diabetes*. 2014:n/a - n/a. doi:10.1111/pedi.12246.

[35] Kuppermann N, Park J, Glatter K, Marcin JP, Glaser NS. Prolonged QT interval corrected for heart rate during diabetic ketoacidosis in children. *Arch. Pediatr Adolesc. Med*. 2008;162(6):544-549.

[36] Kale T, Agrawal H, Pandit R, Naheed Z. T-Wave Inversion in Diabetic Ketoacidosis with Normokalemia in an Adolescent. *Pediatr Cardiol*. 2013;34(6):1508-1510. doi:10.1007/s00246-012-0411-8.

[37] Kutlu AO, Kara C, Cetinkaya S. Rhabdomyolysis without detectable myoglobulinuria due to severe hypophosphatemia in diabetic ketoacidosis. *Pediatr Emerg. Care*. 2011;27(6):537-538.

[38] Haddad NG, Croffie JM, Eugster EA. Pancreatic enzyme elevations in children with diabetic ketoacidosis. *J. Pediatr*. 2004;145(1):122-124. doi:10.1016/j.jpeds.2004.03.050.

[39] Lutfi R, Huang J, Wong HR. Plasmapheresis to Treat Hypertriglyceridemia in a Child With Diabetic Ketoacidosis and Pancreatitis. *PEDIATRICS*. 2012;129(1):e195-e198. doi:10.1542/peds.2011-0217.

[40] Wolfgram PM, MacDonald MJ. Severe Hypertriglyceridemia Causing Acute Pancreatitis in a Child with New Onset Type I Diabetes Mellitus

Presenting in Ketoacidosis. *J. Pediatr Intensive Care*. 2013;2(2):77-80. doi:10.3233/PIC-13053.

[41] Kumar MM, Poovazhagi V, Anbalagan S, Devasena N. Rhino-orbito-cerebral mucormycosis in a child with diabetic ketoacidosis. *Indian J. Crit. Care Med*. 2014;18(5):334-335. doi:10.4103/0972-5229.132512.

[42] Nithyanadam, Ms J, Rr B, Rk T, Ma C, O D. Rhino-Orbito-Cerebral Mucormycosis. A Retrospective Analysis of Clinical Features and Treatment Outcomes. *Indian J. Ophthalmol*. 2003;51(3):231.

[43] Holsclaw DS, Torcato B. Acute pulmonary edema in juvenile diabetic ketoacidosis. *Pediatr Pulmonol*. 1997;24(6):438-443. doi:10.1002/(SICI)1099-0496(199712)24:6<438::AID-PPUL9>3.0.CO;2-C.

[44] Hershey T, Perantie DC, Warren SL, Zimmerman EC, Sadler M, White NH. Frequency and Timing of Severe Hypoglycemia Affects Spatial Memory in Children With Type 1 Diabetes. *Diabetes Care*. 2005;28(10):2372-2377. doi:10.2337/diacare.28.10.2372.

[45] Perantie DC, Lim A, Wu J, et al. Effects of prior hypoglycemia and hyperglycemia on cognition in children with type 1 diabetes mellitus. *Pediatr Diabetes*. 2008;9(2):87-95. doi:10.1111/j.1399-5448.2007.00274.x.

[46] Hershey T, Lillie R, Sadler M, White NH. A prospective study of severe hypoglycemia and long-term spatial memory in children with type 1 diabetes. *Pediatr Diabetes*. 2004;5(2):63-71. doi:10.1111/j.1399-543X.2004.00045.x.

[47] Ghetti S, Lee JK, Sims CE, DeMaster DM, Glaser NS. Diabetic Ketoacidosis and Memory Dysfunction in Children with Type 1 Diabetes. *J. Pediatr*. 2010;156(1):109-114. doi:10.1016/ j.jpeds. 2009.07.054.

[48] Cameron FJ, Scratch SE, Nadebaum C, et al. Neurological Consequences of Diabetic Ketoacidosis at Initial Presentation of Type 1 Diabetes in a Prospective Cohort Study of Children. *Diabetes Care*. 2014;37(6):1554-1562. doi:10.2337/dc13-1904.

In: Pediatric Diabetic Ketoacidosis ISBN: 978-1-63483-220-5
Editors: S. C. Duck and J. R. Hageman

Chapter 7

PEDIATRIC HYPERGLYCEMIC HYPEROSMOLAR STATE

Uchechi Oddiri MD*[1]*, Jaclyn Walsh, MD*[1]*,
***Joseph Hageman, MD,*[1,2] *and Stephen C. Duck, MD*[2]**
[1]University of Chicago Medicine Comer Children's Hospital, Chicago, IL, US
[2]NorthShore University HealthSystem, Evanston, IL, US

ABSTRACT

Unlike Diabetic Ketoacidosis, which has been well described in pediatric literature, Pediatric Hyperglycemic Hyperosmolar State has not been discussed as extensively in current literature, as it is relatively new to pediatrics. This chapter aims to shed light on this disease process as it pertains to the pediatric population. Beginning with the presentation of a patient's case, we will discuss in detail Hyperglycemic Hyperosmolar State's history in medicine, epidemiology, pathophysiology, diagnosis, management recommendations, and complications documented in the pediatric population.

INTRODUCTION

Case Presentation

A 12 year old female with past medical history of obesity and obstructive sleep apnea and no previous diagnosis of diabetes mellitus presented to the emergency department with nausea, vomiting, and diarrhea for 5 days. Her review of systems was positive for: tactile fever, sick contacts with gastroenteritis, and increasing lethargy and sleepiness for 1 day. Her initial vital signs included: weight of 88 kg, body-mass index of 33.1 (95th %tile), temperature of 35.8°C, blood pressure of 89/48 mmHg, heart rate of 102 beats per minute, respiratory rate 30 breaths per minute, and 100% oxygen saturation on room air. Her exam was significant for altered mental status (responsive to tactile stimulus and intermittently to verbal stimuli) and Kussmaul breathing. Initial laboratory findings were significant for: venous blood gas with pH of 6.93, pCO_2 of 25 mmHg, pO_2 of 42 mmHg, and HCO_3^- unable to detect; sodium of 129 mEq/L, potassium (hemolyzed) of 3.5 mEq/L, bicarbonate of < 5 mEq/L, blood urea nitrogen 20 mg/dL, creatinine of 2.4 mg/dL, glucose of 1003 mg/dL. Her serum beta-hydroxybutyrate level was 10.72 mmol/L, serum osmolality 345 mOsm/kg, C-peptide < 0.03 pmol/ml, and Hgb A_1C was 14.6%. Computed tomography image of her head was performed and was negative for acute intracranial process. She was started on maintenance intravenous (IV) fluids, IV regular insulin continuous infusion, and received 1.5L total IVF boluses within the first 24 hours of her presentation to the hospital. With her mental status, mannitol 25g was administered. Over the remainder of her hospital course, her fluid deficit, hyperosmolar diabetic ketoacidosis (DKA), and cerebral edema were managed.

Historical Perspective and Epidemiology

Hyperglycemic Hyperosmolar State (HHS) was described as early as 1886 in a British lecture by Dreschfeld, who noted diabetic coma in patients lacking dyspnea, the scent of acetone on the breath, and acetone or aceto-acetic acid in the urine [1]. The subsequent description in 1957 by Sament and Schwarzis often recognized as the original and, detailed the case of a 32 year old thin male with new onset diabetes. Going forward, most reports of HHS focused on elderly patients with prior type 2 diabetes [1]. The term HHS has been used for over a decade, but other names for the entity, including hyperglycemic coma, hyperosmolar nonketotic coma or state, and diabetic hyperosmolar state had previously been used in the literature to describe a similar constellation of clinical findings.

While it is true that HHS was historically described in adult patients with type 2 diabetes and is still seen with greater incidence in adults, growing rates of pediatric obesity and type 2 diabetes have likely contributed to an increased incidence of HHS in the pediatric population. During the years 1966 to 2001, there were 26 reported cases in the literature, and that number increased to 65 from 2001 to 2008 [1]. It is estimated that up to 4% of children diagnosed with type 2 diabetes present with HHS [2]. Current literature describes as typical characteristics of pediatric HHS patients: male gender, African American race, obese, presence of acanthosis nigricans, family history of diabetes, and poor social network [1, 3-5]. Additionally, infants and children with cognitive impairment, who may be predisposed to dehydration given reduced access to fluids, are at greater risk for HHS [6] (Table 1). Notably, while in the adult population, HHS usually occurs in elderly, malnourished women [7-8], but in children it typically affects previously healthy individuals [9].

Medical literature describing HHS in the pediatric population is still relatively sparse and somewhat limited, but current data estimates pediatric HHS fatality rates of 12-14% [2-3]. This high fatality rate is alarming and could possibly be due to a delay in diagnosis and treatment [5]. Serious complications related to HHS were described in pediatric patients, including cerebral edema, acute renal failure, ventricular arrhythmias, hyperthermia [5], multisystem organ failure [3], pulmonary embolism [10], and rhabdomyolysis [11], typically in patients with irreversible shock and inadequate fluid resuscitation [12] (Table 2).

Table 1. Characteristics of Pediatric HHS Patients

African American race
Family history of diabetes
Male gender
Poor social network
Presence of acanthosis nigrans

Table 2. Serious Complications Related to Pediatrics HHS Patients

Acute renal failure
Cerebral edema
Hyperthermia
Multisystem organ failure
Pulmonary embolism
Rhabdomyolysis
Ventricular arrhythmia
Hypercoagulability/Venous thrombosis

PATHOPHYSIOLOGY

The pathophysiology of HHS is similar to that of DKA but with important key differences. In both HHS and DKA, a marked reduction in the action of circulating insulin [1, 13] (whether due to an actual insulin deficiency or insulin resistance) results in a state of intracellular starvation, which in turn stimulates the release of several counter regulatory hormones, including glucagon, cortisol, catecholamines, and growth hormone [1, 13]. The action of these hormones results in hyperglycemia due to poor glucose utilization by insulin-dependent tissues and increased hepatic and renal glucose production. In DKA, this counter regulatory hormonal response in the face of critically low insulin levels results in subsequent lipolysis and ketogenesis [6]. In HHS, however, individuals typically maintain some low level of insulin that, while insufficient to suppress hepatic glucose production or promote glucose utilization in insulin-dependent tissues, is able to prevent lipolysis and ketogenesis. As a result, HHS patients can have severe hyperglycemia without ketosis or acidosis [1, 5-6, 13]. Some HHS patients, however, present with severe ketoacidosis [9]. These patients hence have mixed DKA and HHS, known as hyperosmolar DKA. In the clinical case [see above], the patient had concomitant ketoacidosis, and hence presented with mixed DKA and HHS.

Apart from hormonal control, an altered renal response is also paramount to the pathogenesis of HHS. Unlike DKA, where the excretion of urinary cations is necessary to balance the excretion of ketoanions, ketosis is not generally present in HHS, so initial electrolyte losses in the urine are reduced as compared to free water losses. Loss of free water worsens hyperosmolarity, resulting in osmotic diuresis and dehydration. Renal function becomes impaired as a result of severe dehydration, which leads to diminished glucose excretion and worsening hyperglycemia [6]. While initial electrolyte losses may be less in HHS than DKA, patients tend to present later and have a longer duration of osmotic diuresis, so there are ultimately more profound electrolyte deficits in HHS [1, 4, 6]. When considering why HHS patients present later than DKA patients, one must recognize that they often have polyuria and polydipsia that increases slowly over time. As such, their symptoms may go unrecognized for a longer period than patients with typical DKA symptoms such as emesis, hyperventilation, and abdominal pain [9].

In the hyperosmolar state, hypertonicity preserves intravascular volume, which masks the previously described profound dehydration [1, 4]. Fluid resuscitation causes a decrease in serum osmolality, which results in decreased intravascular volume as water moves from intravascular to intracellular/interstitial spaces via an osmotic gradient [1]. With treatment, patients also undergo significant osmotic diuresis, so their fluid requirements can be massive in order to reverse shock and avoid severe complications of HHS [14].

Diagnosis

The criteria to establish a diagnosis of HHS include [15]:

- A plasma glucose concentration of 600 mg/dL or greater
- Venous pH > 7.25; arterial pH > 7.30*
- Serum bicarbonate > 15 mmol/L*
- Small ketonuria, absent to mild ketonemia*
- Serum osmolality > 320 mOsm/kg
- Altered mental status or seizures.

[*Except in cases with mixed DKA and HHS, otherwise known as hyperosmolar DKA.]

In patients with mixed DKA and HHS, or hyperosmolar DKA, moderate to severe ketosis and acidemia can be present [9]. In the clinical case [see above], the patient presented with characteristics of DKA (with pH of 6.93, bicarbonate < 5 mg/dL, glucose 1003 mg/dL, and beta-hydroxybutyrate 10.72 mmol/L), as well as those of HHS (glucose 1003 mg/dL, serum osmolality 345 mOsm/kg, and altered mentation). This placed the patient into the hyperosmolar DKA category.

Management

There are distinct differences in the management of DKA, HHS, and mixed cases, also known as Hyperosmolar DKA (Figure 1). There are no prospective data to guide treatment of HHS in the pediatric population. The following recommendations are per the Consensus Statement from the International Society for Pediatric and Adolescent Diabetes [15]:

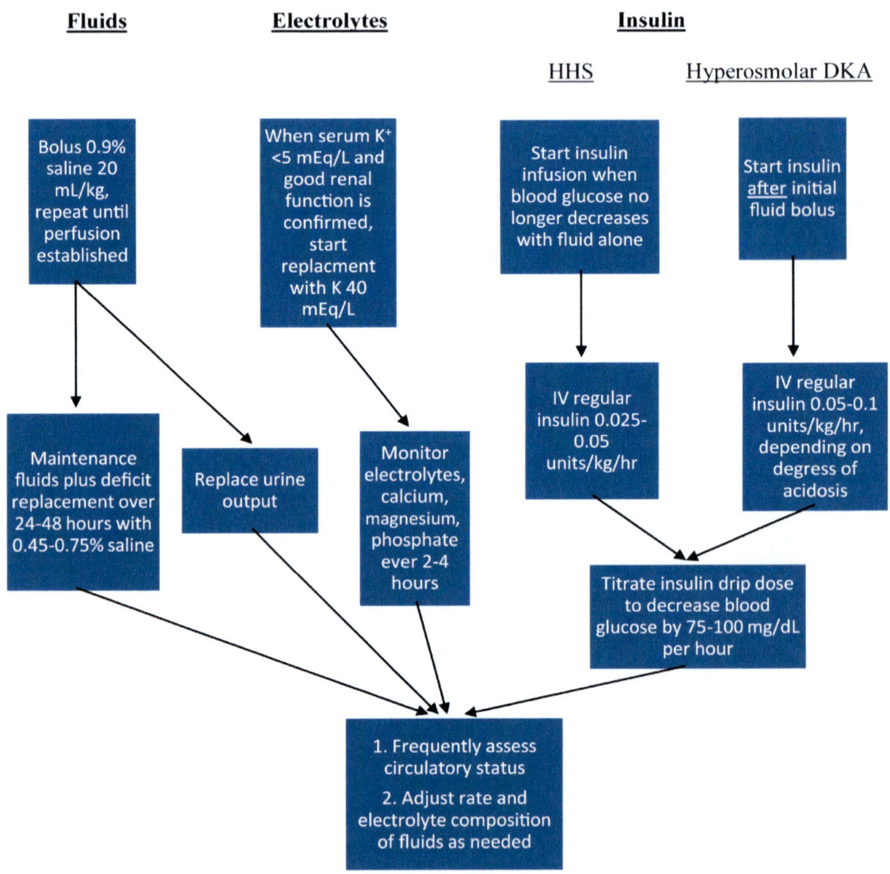

Figure 1. Treatment of Hyperglycemic Hyperosmolar State (HHS) in children. Adapted from Zeitler et al. [23].

1. Assess Patient's Airway

(a) Establish their Glasgow Coma Scale if mental status is altered. If needed, secure the airway and decompress the stomach with a nasogastric tube.
(b) Avoid intubation if possible, as it may lead to rapid increase in pCO2 during the intubation process, which may cause a decrease in cerebrospinal fluid pH and worsen existing cerebral edema [16].
(c) For a patient who recently ingested a large volume of fruit juice or sweetened soft drinks, consider emptying the stomach even if the patient is not obtunded to avoid further absorption of glucose and electrolyte-free water from the intestinal tract [17-18].
(d) If patient demonstrates signs or symptoms of cerebral edema (headache, bradycardia, hypertension, altered mental status, focal findings on neurological exam, hypoxemia), please proceed with management for cerebral edema (further described below).

2. Fluid Therapy

With the larger amount of fluid loss in HHS compared to DKA, fluid therapy in HHS aims to replete this volume. Identifying the degree of dehydration can be difficult among the obese and because the hypertonicity in HHS preserves the intravascular volume.

(a) Initial bolus of ≥20 mL/kg of isotonic saline should be given and repeated as needed to restore normal renal perfusion.
(b) Once normal renal perfusion has been restored, hypernatremia may be addressed with 0.45-0.75% saline to replete free water deficit. The goal is to gradually correct serum sodium and osmolality.
(c) If corrected sodium concentration fails to reduce with treatment, this may be an indication for dialysis. In this situation, hemodialysis was associated with 80% survival as opposed to 20% survival with peritoneal dialysis [1]. The recommended rate of drop of sodium concentration is 0.5 mmol/L/hour [19].
(d) With volume repletion alone (prior to initiating insulin therapy), blood glucose should decrease by 75-100 mg/dL/hour due to the improved renal perfusion and resulting glucosuria [20-21]. A more rapid decline necessitates 2.5 or 5% dextrose to be added to rehydration fluid.

Failure of blood glucose concentration to decline during rehydration should prompt reassessment and evaluation of renal function. In these cases, insulin therapy may be necessary.

(e) Replacement of renal fluid volume losses is recommended [22].

3. Insulin

(a) Unless there is a mixed presentation with HHS and DKA, ketosis in HHS is usually minimal at the most. The serum glucose should decline with rehydration fluid therapy at a rate of 50-100 mg/dL/hour. If it fails to do so, insulin therapy should be initiated. In patients with more severe ketoacidosis, insulin therapy should be initiated sooner [9].

(b) IV regular insulin should be started at 0.025-0.05 units/kg/hour and titrated to achieve decline in serum glucose by 50-75 mg/dL/hour.

(c) Insulin boluses are not recommended.

4. Electrolytes

a. Potassium
   (i) As soon as serum potassium concentration is within normal range and patient has adequate urine output, potassium supplementation should be initiated with at least 40 mmol/L of replacement fluid.
   (ii) Serum potassium concentration should be monitor every 2-3 hours, and more frequently if patient is hypokalemic.

b. Bicarbonate therapy is not recommended.

c. Phosphate
   (i) Phosphate repletion is recommended as hypophosphatemia may lead to rhabdomyolysis, hemolytic uremia, muscle weakness, and paralysis.
   (ii) Using an IV solution with 50:50 mixture of potassium phosphate and another potassium salt (potassium chloride or potassium acetate) repletes phosphate without inducing hypocalcemia.

d. Magnesium
   (i) Although hypomagnesemia has been noted in patients with HHS, no study has shown that magnesium repletion is beneficial.

(ii) Magnesium repletion may be considered in a patient with severe hypomagnesemia and hypocalcemia. The recommended dose is 25–50 mg/kg per dose for 3–4 doses given every 4–6 h with a maximum infusion rate of 150 mg/min and 2 g/h [15].

COMPLICATIONS

1. Cerebral Edema

Studies of chronic hypertonicity suggest that brain cells produce osmotically active substances, "idiogenic osmoles," that preserve intracellular osmolality, and hence intracellular volume [23-26]. Therefore, it is theorized that pediatric patients with HHS with prolonged hypertonicity are at greater risk for cerebral edema than those with DKA. Also, patients are believed to be at risk for cerebral edema if the rate of decline in serum osmolality exceeds the rate at which neurons can eliminate the idiogenic osmoles [9].

Cerebral edema usually becomes clinically evident with the first 12 hours after initiation of treatment, but can occur before treatment has started [27-28] or as late as 24-48 hours after the initiation of treatment [29]. Signs and symptoms of cerebral edema include: headache, hypertension, bradycardia, change in neurological status, localizing neurological deficits on exam, and hypoxemia. Muir et al., [30] developed a clinical assessment tool for the diagnosis of cerebral edema in children following initiation of their therapy [see below]. The presence of one diagnostic criterion, or two major criteria, or one major and two minor criteria have a sensitivity of 92% and a false positive rate of 4%.

Diagnostic Criteria

a. Abnormal motor or verbal response to pain
b. Decorticate or decerebrate posture
c. Cranial nerve palsy (especially III, IV, and VI)
d. Abnormal neurogenic respiratory pattern (e.g., grunting tachypnea, Cheyne-Stokes respiration, apneusis)

Major Criteria

a. Altered or fluctuating mental status
b. Sustained heart rate deceleration (decrease more than 20 beats/min) not attributable to improved fluid resuscitation or sleep state
c. Age-inappropriate incontinence

Minor Criteria

a. Vomiting
b. Headache
c. Lethargy or difficulty to arouse
d. Diastolic blood pressure > 90 mmHg
e. Age < 5 years

Treatment of cerebral edema should begin as soon as it is suspected. Fluid administration should be reduced by one third [15]. Hypertonic solution (mannitol or hypertonic 3% saline) should be used. Mannitol is dosed 0.5-1 g/kg IV over 10-15 minutes and repeated if no initial response is noted after 30 minutes to 2 hours [31]. Hypertonic saline (3%) may be dosed 2.5-5 mL/kg over 10-15 minutes and may be used as an alternative to mannitol [32-33]. Head of bed should be elevated to 30°. Intubate as necessary. After treatment for cerebral edema has been initiated, head imaging may be considered to determine if patient has a lesion requiring neurosurgical intervention (e.g, intracranial hemorrhage) or a lesion that may necessitate anticoagulation (e.g., cerebrovascular thrombosis) [34-37].

2. Venous Thrombosis/Hypercoagulability

Venous thrombosis is a common complication when central venous catheters are used in HHS patients [38]. No data has indicated benefit in using prophylactic low-dose heparin. Heparin treatment is recommended for children with HHS who require central venous catheters and are immobile for > 24-48 hours [9].

3. Rhabdomyolysis

The clinical signs of rhabdomyolysis include weakness, myalgia, and dark urine [15]. Rhabdomyolysis may occur in children with HHS resulting in acute renal injury, severe hyperkalemia, hypocalcemia, and muscle swelling (sometimes causing compartment syndrome) [39]. Creatine kinase concentrations should be monitored every 2-3 hours for early detection [15].

4. Malignant Hyperthermia

Malignant hyperthermia is of unknown etiology in children with HHS, but is consistent with a high mortality rate. A patient with a fever and elevated creatine kinase concentration may be treated with dantrolene. However, only one of three pediatric patients with HHS treated with dantrolene survived [10-11,40].

REFERENCES

[1] Rosenbloom, AL. Hyperglycemic hyperosmolar state: an emerging pediatric problem. *J Pediatr*, 2010, 156, 180–184.

[2] Fourtner S. Hyperglycemic hyperosmolar nonketotic syndrome in children. *Proc Endocr Soc 85th Annual Meeting*. Philadelphia, PA; 2003. Abstract OR42-46.

[3] Fourtner, SH; Weinzimer, SA; Levitt Katz, LE. Hyperglycemic hyperosmolar non-ketotic syndrome in children with type 2 diabetes. *Pediatr Diabetes*. 2005, 6,129-135.

[4] Bassham, B; Estrada, C; Abramo, T. Hyperglycemic hyperosmolar syndrome in the pediatric patient. *Pediatric Emergency Care*. 2012, 28, 699-702.

[5] Cochran, JB; Walters, S; Losek, JD. Pediatric hyperglycemic hyperosmolar syndrome: diagnostic difficulties and high mortality rate. *Am J Emerg Med*. 2006, 24, 297-301.

[6] Glaser, N. Pediatric diabetic ketoacidosis and hyperglycemic hyperosmolar state. *Pediatr Clin North Am*. 2005, 52, 1611-1635·

[7] Wachtel, TJ; Silliman, RA; Lamberton, P. Predisposing factors for the diabetic hyperosmolar state. *Arch Intern Med*. 1987, 147, 499-501.

[8] Wang, J; Williams, DE; Narayan, KM. Declining death rates from hyperglycemic crisis among adults with diabetes, U.S., 1985-2002. *Diabetes Care*. 2006, 29, 2018-2022.

[9] Zeitler, P; Haqq, A; Rosenbloom, A; Glaser, N. Hyperglycemic hyperosmolar syndrome in children: pathophysiological considerations and suggested guidelines for treatment. *J Pediatr*, 2011, 158, 9–14, 14 e11–12.

[10] Morales, AE; Rosenbloom, AL. Death caused by hyperglycemic hyperosmolar state at the onset of type 2 diabetes. *J Pediatr*, 2004, 144, 270–273.
[11] Hollander, AS; Olney, RC; Blackett, PR; Marshall, BA. Fatal malignant hyperthermia-like syndrome with rhabdomyolysis complicating the presentation of diabetes mellitus in adolescent males. *Pediatrics*, 2003, 111 (6 Pt 1), 1447–1452.
[12] Canerie, MF; Bogue, CW; Banasiak, KJ; et al. Decompensated hyperglycemic hyperosmolarity without significant ketoacidosis in the adolescent and young adult population. *J Pediatr Endocrinol Metab*. 2007, 10, 1115-1124.
[13] Rosenbloom, AL. Hyperglycemic comas in children: new insights into pathophysiology and management. *Rev Endocr Metab Disord*. 2005, 6, 297-306.
[14] Kitabchi, AE; Umpierrez, GE; Miles, JM; et al. Hyperglycemic crises in adult patients with diabetes. *Diabetes Care*. 2009, 7, 1335-1343.
[15] Wolfsdorf, JI; Allgrove, J; Craig, ME; Edge, J; Glaser, N; Jain, V; Lee, WWR; Mungai, LNW; Rosenbloom, AL; Sperling, MA; Hanas, R. A Consensus Statement from the International Society for Pediatric and Adolescent Diabetes: Diabetic ketoacidosis and hyperglycemic hyperosmolar state. *Pediatric Diabetes*, 2014, 15 (Suppl. 20): 154–179.
[16] Tasker, RC; Lutman, D; Peters, MJ. Hyperventilation in severe diabetic ketoacidosis. *Pediatr Crit Care Med*, 2005, 6, 405–411.
[17] Carlotti, AP; St George-Hyslop, C; Guerguerian, AM; Bohn, D; Kamel, KS; Halperin, M. Occult risk factor for the development of cerebral edema in children with diabetic ketoacidosis: possible role for stomach emptying. *Pediatr Diabetes*, 2009, 10, 522–533.
[18] Davids, MR; Edoute, Y; Stock, S; Halperin, ML. Severe degree of hyperglycaemia: insights from integrative Physiology. *QJM*, 2002, 95, 113–124.
[19] Kronan, K; Normal, ME. Renal and electrolyte emergencies. In: Fleisher GR, Ludwig S, eds. Textbook of Emergency Medicine. 4th edn. Philadelphia: Lippincott Williams and Wilkins, 2000.
[20] Matz, R. Management of the hyperosmolar hyperglycemic syndrome. *Am Fam Physician*, 1999, 60, 1468–1476.
[21] Delaney, MF; Zisman, A; Kettyle, WM. Diabetic ketoacidosis and hyperglycemic hyperosmolar nonketotic syndrome. *Endocrinol Metab Clin North Am*, 2000, 29, 683–705, V.

[22] Kitabchi, AE; Umpierrez, GE; Fisher, JN; Murphy, MB; Stentz, FB. Thirty years of personal experience in hyperglycemic crises: diabetic ketoacidosis and hyperglycemic hyperosmolar state. *J Clin Endocrinol Metab*, 2008, 93, 1541–1552.

[23] Rosenbloom, AL. Hyperglycemic crises and their complications in children. *J Pediatr Endocrinol Metab*, 2007, 20,5-18.

[24] Goldman, SL. Hyperglycemic hyperosmolar coma in a 9-month-old child. *Am J Dis Child*, 1979, 133,181-3.

[25] Gordon, EE; Kabadi, UM. The hyperglycemic hyperosmolar syndrome. *Am J Med Sci*, 1976, 271,252-68.

[26] Conley, S. Hypernatremia. *Pediatr Clin North Am*, 1990, 37,365-72.

[27] Glaser, N; Barnett, P; McCaslin, I; et al. Risk factors for cerebral edema in children with diabetic ketoacidosis. The Pediatric Emergency Medicine Collaborative Research Committee of the American Academy of Pediatrics. *N Engl J Med*, 2001, 344, 264–269.

[28] Deeb, L. Development of fatal cerebral edema during outpatient therapy for diabetic ketoacidosis. *Pract Diabetes*, 1989, 6, 212–213.

[29] Rosenbloom, AL. Intracerebral crises during treatment of diabetic ketoacidosis. *Diabetes Care*, 1990, 13, 22–33.

[30] Muir, AB; Quisling, RG; Yang, MC; Rosenbloom, AL. Cerebral edema in childhood diabetic ketoacidosis: natural history, radiographic findings, and early identification. *Diabetes Care*, 2004, 27, 1541–1546.

[31] Franklin, B; Liu, J; Ginsberg-Fellner, F. Cerebral edema and ophthalmoplegia reversed by mannitol in a new case of insulin-dependent diabetes mellitus. *Pediatrics*, 1982, 69, 87–90.

[32] Curtis, JR; Bohn, D; Daneman, D. Use of hypertonic saline in the treatment of cerebral edema in diabetic ketoacidosis (DKA). *Pediatr Diabetes*, 2001, 2, 191–194.

[33] Kamat, P; Vats, A; Gross, M; Checchia, PA. Use of hypertonic saline for the treatment of altered mental status associated with diabetic ketoacidosis. *Pediatr Crit Care Med*, 2003, 4, 239–242.

[34] Keane, S; Gallagher, A; Ackroyd, S; McShane, MA; Edge, JA. Cerebral venous thrombosis during diabetic ketoacidosis. *Arch Dis Child*, 2002, 86, 204–205.

[35] Kanter, RK; Oliphant, M; Zimmerman, JJ; Stuart, MJ. Arterial thrombosis causing cerebral edema in association with diabetic ketoacidosis. *Crit Care Med*, 1987, 15, 175–176.

[36] Roe, TF; Crawford, TO; Huff, KR; Costin, G; Kaufman, FR; Nelson, MD; Jr. Brain infarction in children with diabetic ketoacidosis. *J Diabetes Complications*, 1996, 10, 100–108.

[37] Rosenbloom, AL. Fatal cerebral infarctions in diabetic ketoacidosis in a child with previously unknown heterozygosity for factor V Leiden deficiency. *J Pediatr*, 2004, 145, 561–562.

[38] Gutierrez, JA; Bagatell, R; Samson, MP; Theodorou, AA; Berg, RA. Femoral central venous catheter associated deep venous thrombosis in children with diabetic ketoacidosis. *Crit Care Med*, 2003, 31, 80–83.

[39] Hollander, AS; Olney, RC; Blackett, PR; Marshall, BA. Fatal malignant hyperthermia-like syndrome with rhabdomyolysis complicating the presentation of diabetes mellitus in adolescent males. *Pediatrics*, 2003, 111 (6 Pt 1), 1447–1452.

[40] Kilbane, BJ; Mehta, S; Backeljauw, PF; Shanley, TP; Crimmins, NA. Approach to management of malignant hyperthermia-like syndrome in pediatric diabetes mellitus. *Pediatr Crit Care Med*, 2006, 7, 169–173.

EDITORS' CONTACT INFORMATION

Dr. Stephen Duck, MD
Pediatric Endroconologist, Department of Pediatrics
NorthShore University HealthSystem,
Evanston, Il. 6021 Senior Clinician Educator
Prtizker School of Medicine
University of Chicago, Chicago, Il
Email: sduck@northshore.org

Joseph R. Hageman, MD
Emeritus Attending Pediatrician Department of Pediatrics
NorthShore University HealthSystem
Evanston, Il. Senior Clinician Educator
Prtizker School of Medicine
University of Chicago, Chicago, Il
Email: jhageman@peds.bsd.uchicago.edu

INDEX

H

I

K

L

M

O